teach®
yourself

reflexology
chris stormer

teach yourself
70
celebrate
with us

Launched in 1938, the **teach yourself** series grew rapidly in response to the world's wartime needs. Loved and trusted by over 50 million readers, the series has continued to respond to society's changing interests and passions and now, 70 years on, includes over 500 titles, from Arabic and Beekeeping to Yoga and Zulu. What would you like to learn?

be where you want to be with **teach yourself**

For UK order enquiries: please contact Bookpoint Ltd, 130 Milton Park, Abingdon, Oxon, OX14 4SB. Telephone: +44 (0) 1235 827720. Fax: +44 (0) 1235 400454. Lines are open 09.00–17.00, Monday to Saturday, with a 24-hour message answering service. Details about our titles and how to order are available at www.teachyourself.co.uk

For USA order enquiries: please contact McGraw-Hill Customer Services, PO Box 545, Blacklick, OH 43004-0545, USA. Telephone: 1-800-722-4726. Fax: 1-614-755-5645.

For Canada order enquiries: please contact McGraw-Hill Ryerson Ltd, 300 Water St, Whitby, Ontario, L1N 9B6, Canada. Telephone: 905 430 5000. Fax: 905 430 5020.

Long renowned as the authoritative source for self-guided learning – with more than 50 million copies sold worldwide – the **teach yourself** series includes over 500 titles in the fields of languages, crafts, hobbies, business, computing and education.

British Library Cataloguing in Publication Data: a catalogue record for this title is available from the British Library.

Library of Congress Catalog Card Number: on file.

First published in UK 1996 by Hodder Education, part of Hachette Live UK, 338 Euston Road, London, NW1 3BH.

First published in US 1996 by The McGraw-Hill Companies, Inc.

This edition published 2007.

The **teach yourself** name is a registered trade mark of Hodder Headline.

Typeset by Transet Limited, Coventry, England.
Printed in Great Britain for Hodder Education, an Hachette Livre UK Company, 338 Euston Road, London NW1 3BH, by Cox & Wyman Ltd, Reading, Berkshire.

The publisher has used its best endeavours to ensure that the URLs for external websites referred to in this book are correct and active at the time of going to press. However, the publisher and the author have no responsibility for the websites and can make no guarantee that a site will remain live or that the content will remain relevant, decent or appropriate.

Hachette Livre UK's policy is to use papers that are natural, renewable and recyclable products and made from wood grown in sustainable forests. The logging and manufacturing processes are expected to conform to the environmental regulations of the country of origin.

Impression number   10 9 8 7 6 5 4 3
Year   2010 2009

contents

acknowledgements		**xi**
introduction		**xiii**
01	**reflexology at a glance**	**1**
	a brief explanation	2
	ongoing benefits	3
	advantages of learning reflexology	3
	background	4
	worshipping feet	5
	the relief of it all	5
02	**a complementary art of healing**	**7**
	modern medicine and reflexology	8
	teaming up together	8
	lifestyle changes	9
	other complementary steps	9
03	**ease or 'dis-ease'**	**11**
	your approach to life	12
	re-assessing your life	12
	disturbing your status quo	13
	reflexology steps in	14
	signs that all is not well	15
	the remedy at hand	15
04	**who benefits from reflexology?**	**16**
	in pregnancy	17
	babies and children	17
	teenagers	18
	adults	18
	seniors	19

distressed souls 19

the family unit 20

05 **a closer look at reflexology** **21**

let your feet speak 22

the condition of your soles 22

literally 'at your feet' 22

get ahead through your feet 23

how reflexology works 23

from the inside out 25

a powerful relaxation technique 25

06 **body reflections** **26**

ongoing knowledge 27

picture your body on your feet 28

out on your limbs 31

either side 32

07 **the power of your touch** **33**

the importance of touch 34

making contact 34

healing through your hands 35

for the best results 35

give credit where it's due 36

08 **foot characteristics** **37**

take a closer look 38

colour 39

left and right 39

angle 40

09 **your state of mind** **41**

brain reflexes 42

toepads 42

toe by toe 43

brain, hair and sinuses 44

forehead and midbrain 45

back of head and neck 46

belief systems 46

your state of mind 47

10	**toe characteristics**	**48**
	shape	49
	size	49
	skin	49
11	**your back and neck**	**51**
	spine	52
	the arches of your feet	53
	nerves	53
	hands	54
	feet	55
	complete inner calm	56
12	**your big toes and toe necks**	**57**
	your 'thoughtful' big toes	58
	keeping your hormones in check	59
	sensory system	60
13	**your expressive parts**	**62**
	throat	63
	neck	63
	neck and throat problems	64
	thyroid gland	65
	shoulders	66
	wrists	66
	ankles	67
	so what do you think?	68
14	**your second toes and the balls of your feet**	**69**
	your second 'feeling' toes	70
	emotions	71
	eyes	72
	your insightful inner tutor	72
	the balls of your feet	73
	fluctuating emotions	74
	lungs	75
	breathing and respiratory problems	76
	breast reflexes	76
	thymus gland	77

	oesophagus	78
	airways	79
	elbows	79
	knees	80
	solar plexus	81
	ribs	82
	lower arms	82
	shins	83
	upper thoracic vertebrae	83
	liberating the breath	84
	your heart	84
	blood and circulation	85
15	**your third toes and the upper halves of your insteps**	**87**
	your third 'doing' toes	88
	nose	89
	ears	90
	cheeks	91
	digestion	91
	liver	92
	gall bladder	93
	pancreas	94
	spleen	95
	adrenal glands	96
	cardiac sphincter	97
	stomach	98
	pyloric sphincter	99
	duodenum	99
	jejunum	100
	middle back	101
	getting on with your life	101
16	**your fourth toes and lower portions of your insteps**	**103**
	your fourth 'relationship' toes	104
	mouth	105
	small intestine	106

ileo-caecal valve   107

appendix   108

bowels   109

female reproductive organs   110

ovaries   110

fallopian tubes   111

kidneys   112

ureter   113

upper arms   113

lumber vertebrae   114

digestive process   115

17   **your little toes and heels**   **116**

family and social belief systems   117

heels   118

jaw   118

skin   119

skeleton   119

muscles   120

pelvic bone   121

hips   122

buttocks   122

rectum   123

anus   124

bladder   124

urethra   125

lower reproductive parts   126

uterus   127

vagina   127

male reproductive organs   128

testes   129

the base of your back   129

18   **pregnancy**   **131**

before conception   132

during pregnancy   132

during childbirth   134

after childbirth   135

19   **the technique**   **136**

four simple movements   137

technique 1 – rotation   137

technique 2 – caterpillar   138

technique 3 – stroking or milking   138

technique 4 – feathering or healing caress   139

20   **what to expect**   **141**

the sensations experienced   142

less common reactions   142

pleasurable after-effects   143

excellent signs of healing   143

unusual reactions   144

21   **preparing for the reflexology massage**   **146**

preparation   147

communication   148

comfort   149

helpful reminder   149

22   **reflexology step by step**   **151**

the warm-up   152

soothe the nerves   160

open the avenues of expression   167

re-establish a firm backbone   172

the metamorphic technique   176

harmonize the endocrine system   178

take in the breath of life   184

restore the digestive system   187

re-energize the whole system   190

re-instate the bones, muscles and skin   202

restrengthening the limbs   203

appease the reproductive organs   208

release the past   211

the finale   213

first-aid reflexology   218

if you are at all concerned   218

23	**a summary of the massage**	**219**
	the sequence	220
	reflexology today and in the future	222
taking it further		**224**
appendix I		**230**
appendix II		**231**
appendix III		**233**
appendix IV		**234**
index		**235**

dedication

In loving memory of my beloved mother
DAPHNE MARIAN CORNER

acknowledgements

To have Hodder Education as my publisher is indeed a privilege, as is the opportunity to re-edit this book, which was first published in 1996. It's fantastic to see how far I have come, and to realize how much more the Universe trusts me to share this amazing information; I am truly blessed.

None of this would have been possible without the incredible love and support of my man, John Fryer! My two wonderful sons, Andrew and David, have long since left home but they still continue to be there for me from a distance, as does my amazing father, Dick Corner. My beloved mother, Daphne Corner, is now an angel, who continues to inspire me from the other side.

I am eternally grateful to Sally Teixeira, Sarisha Harilal and Susanne Mason for stepping in at the last moment to help me out with the editing. Then there's Val Seddon, my 'Astral Mum', who is always on the other end of the telephone, sharing her wisdom whenever it is most needed. Meanwhile, at our divine Good Vibrations Health Sanctuary in Johannesburg, is our lovely Leah Ramaliba, who constantly has a smile on her face as she keeps everything running smoothly.

There are literally thousands of reflexology students, teachers and practitioners worldwide, who have inspired me during the past 20 years, ever since I first became passionate about feet, along with a host of other natural healers, all of whom are very dear to me. Thank you to you all, as well as to the numerous delegates who attend my seminars, for your ongoing faith and encouragement. I am in the fantastic position that I am in today because of you; my heartfelt love and appreciation goes to each and every one of you.

Then to you, dear reader, I honour your decision to take your 'understanding' a step further, because without you, books like this would not be possible.

May you all enjoy abundant happiness and ultimate fulfilment every step of the way.

introduction

Here's the ideal opportunity to finally put your feet up and pamper yourself! With *Teach Yourself Reflexology* by your side, you will be guided, step by step, through this incredibly safe yet extremely effective form of natural healing. It really is an excellent way in which to regain and maintain your health.

There is nothing new about the concept of reflexology, which has been around since humans first set foot on earth, so it has most certainly stood the test of time. It is as effective now as it was then. This book looks back at its origins, a fascinating journey in itself, and shows how, since the beginning of time, reflexology has served humanity as an outstanding and incredible means of encouraging mind, body and soul to heal themselves. The information shared here has been updated to give you an insight into the endless possibilities of this ancient therapy.

Meanwhile, the explicit instructions of how to massage both feet guides you meaningfully, section by section, to reveal how, by taking a weight off your mind, when massaging your toes, you have more space to think; it shows how, by caressing your toe necks, you derive the very best from the two-way exchange of life-force energies that enter and leave your body; it discloses how, by stroking the balls of your feet, your ruffled emotions are soothed and dispensed with; it divulges how, by kneading your insteps, you have the courage to face daily challenges and have much healthier relationships and, finally, it makes sure that, by rubbing your heels, you know how to make the most incredible progress in your life so that you feel so much better about yourself and others.

The great thing about reflexology is that there is no one way of doing it. This means that you can adjust the outlined procedures and develop your own unique approach. Fortunately it is very accommodating and it really *does not matter* if your attempts are initially slow, cumbersome, inaccurate or confused, the body knows exactly what to do and compensates accordingly, so you can relax!

It is impossible to cause harm, even in inexperienced hands.

There are plenty of clear and concise illustrations to assist you in getting to know 'what's afoot'. It really is so fascinating to see how your transient thoughts and inner emotions are constantly mirrored onto your feet and how this insight can be used to know how best to massage feet. You will be amazed at how quickly individuals respond to reflexology, no matter how well or ill they are initially, provided they wish to get better. Even if they don't, there is often a favourable shift to help them change their mind!

The soothing movements of the massage encourage vital mind-shifts, which help pacify inner uneasiness, whilst the caressing movements have the most incredible knack of transforming fraught, uptight individuals into relaxed, easy-going and energized beings. Reflexology is truly remarkable! It encourages you, along with everybody else, to help yourselves to a more fulfilling, rewarding and better way of life. No matter how sceptical you may be initially, the effects of massaging feet are bound to impress you! They can be truly miraculous; so find out for yourself by experiencing it and seeing it in action!

You possess a very great power, the ability to heal yourself!

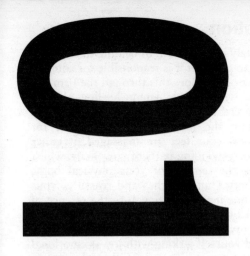

01

reflexology at a glance

In this chapter you will learn:
- how reflexology can help you and others
- about ongoing benefits
- its background and history.

A brief explanation

Reflexology is a completely natural form of healing that is non-evasive, simple and safe to give, yet it is responsible for some of the most impressive reactions. It does this through the firm but gentle massage of feet, which alerts latent healing abilities within your body and creates greater peace and harmony within, thereby providing the most ideal environment for health. As the reflexes on your feet are massaged, it either arouses or soothes the corresponding parts of your body, whilst the massage itself eases the tension of your physical body, quietens your mental chatter, and soothes and reassures your emotions. At the same time it reconnects you to the essence of your spirit. As the welcome surge of vibrant energy rushes through your body, it rejuvenates your whole being to such an extent that you may find yourself jerking with joy as emotional impediments are flushed away. This is followed, almost immediately, by a blissful state of inner peace that washes over you, offering you a much needed respite from the chaos of everyday life.

Reflexology gives you the time and space to sort out your mind and re-establish your priorities.

How reflexology helps

The relaxation aspect of reflexology is important since it is only when you are truly relaxed and at ease with yourself that you are able to determine what is best for you to regain and retain excellent health. When you are not feeling so good, reflexology has much to offer since it relieves discomfort, be it in the form of aches, pains, cramps or whatever is upsetting you. What makes it so effective is that it gets to the very root of a problem, so that the memory associated with it can be sorted out and eliminated once and for all. Its beneficial effects then continue from there: counteracting fatigue, tiredness and exhaustion; soothing nervousness, concern, worry or fear and also alleviating undue distress. In so doing it clears your whole body of impure thoughts and toxic emotions by improving your circulation, and stimulating underactive, sluggish areas so they start working well for you again. It also calms hyperactive, over-productive parts and stops them from draining you.

You feel totally recharged and fit for life!

Ongoing benefits

Once you feel better, reflexology is one of the best ways to stay in tip-top condition, but you do need regular top-ups – ideally once a week – to keep it that way. A one-off session is great for getting you back on your feet, but it is keeping you there that makes the difference. It is such a pleasant form of deep relaxation and gives such welcome relief from daily strains, frustrations and irritations, that it has to be good for you. Receiving it regularly makes sure that you feel constantly rejuvenated and re-energized. Your vitality is increased, your confidence is boosted, you sleep so much better and it enhances your trust in yourself and others. You can then focus on what's important in your life. It gives you such an incredible feeling of well-being that you feel whole again and can enjoy a more fulfilling and rewarding lifestyle. From the very core of your being comes the courage and wisdom to cope with any perceived adversity and the opportunity to present the 'true you'; this in itself brings endless opportunities for ongoing transformation, growth and progress.

Just keep getting better at being yourself!

Advantages of learning reflexology

There are many advantages to learning and giving reflexology, especially since anybody can do it, if they wish to. It can also be given at any time and anywhere, since all you need are your hands and the recipient's feet. Academic achievements are not a prerequisite and medical knowledge is useful but not essential. Furthermore; since only the feet are exposed, there is no embarrassment, self-consciousness or fear of feeling vulnerable. Painful body parts remain undisturbed yet still benefit from the relief when their related reflexes are being massaged. Also, with less skin surface on the feet than on the body, a more thorough and precise treatment is possible.

As you become more adept and familiar with reflexology you will soon realize that it has many far-reaching effects and offers you so much more than just an opportunity to massage feet. It takes you into a whole world that comes with feet; making reflexology a fascinating, enjoyable and rewarding journey during which you come to really understand the intrigues of your own body, mind and spirit.

The massage itself generally takes around an hour, yet its effects last much longer, thanks to reflexology's encompassing and wholistic approach.

Health and healing are only two feet away!

Background

When humans first set foot on earth their soles were naturally stimulated every time they took a step, with the undulating, rocky surfaces keeping them in good shape. That is until sandals and shoes came into being! Footwear immediately created barriers and, in so doing, diminished the feet's innate sensitivity. Today they still keep you 'in the dark', which is why sometimes you have little or no idea of how to adapt to what's going on 'under foot'. Reflexology replaces the impetus that is needed to get you going. The importance of reflexology was acknowledged, even before shoes, by virtually every tribe worldwide and, at one time, was alleged to be everybody's birthright, so much so that youngsters were taught how to do it from a very early age, to ensure that this knowledge was passed on from generation to generation.

Feet have always symbolized mobility and security and are seen to be the foundation of mind, body and soul.

Step back for a moment

According to Greek legend, feet mirror the soul and any lameness was considered to be weakness of spirit, which is possibly why many flocked to a well-known health resort in Delphi until AD200. Here they received reflexology, along with various other spa massages, before retiring to a sleep temple; where memories were evoked to bring the foresight to deal with every day life.

Meanwhile, across the seas, in ancient Egypt, it was believed that the soles kept the soul safe inside the body, which is why during mummification, the bottoms of the feet were peeled away to set the spirit free and release it from its bondage and commitment to earth. A great deal of attention was also given to feet in the Far East, and, according to Japanese mythology, there was a wise old soul called Outo, who, when questioned about his incredible healing abilities would answer: 'See to the feet, my friend, and you have seen the body!' Around this time there was an increasing awareness, worldwide, of witches, who claimed to absorb their mystical powers from the earth through their feet, which terrified the masses so much that as soon as anybody was found guilty of practising witchcraft their feet were immediately lifted from the ground. These are just a few examples of how feet have been viewed, revered and feared.

Remember to use your wisdom, knowledge and experiences to move onto the next stage of your journey through life!

Worshipping feet

In the Bible there are numerous references to the symbolic ritual of welcome and purification through the washing, anointing and massaging of feet. Reflexology is a furtherance of this sacred act since it, too, cleanses the body and creates an inner purity, which is absolutely essential for healing. Today the feet of divine or eminent beings are still kissed and worshipped, as a sign of respect, a practice that was once common in most cultures worldwide. Even now, in certain rural areas of India, youngsters are expected to laud over their parent's feet to show their love and appreciation. Also in India, every year thousands of devotees travel to ashrams throughout the country for the opportunity to glimpse or touch the feet of devout, spiritual men, known as *babas*. These devotees believe it to be their way of achieving eternal peace and personal enlightenment. Other ways in which they do this is by gathering dust from the *baba's* footprints, or drinking water that has been poured over the *baba's* feet.

All religions, arts and sciences are branches of the same tree.

The relief of it all

Feet represent your roots and your foundation. The moment you restrict yourself, you limit your potential and tense your feet, but as soon as you free your mind from self-limiting constraints, your feet relax and you are able to move on unimpeded, which is ancient knowledge. Yet for centuries, many have tried different means of pain relief, but continued to suffer until they discovered reflexology. One of these individuals was the twentieth president of the United States of America,

President Garfield (1831–81), who suffered excruciating pain after an assassination attempt. Despite an endless repertoire of various treatments his pain just wouldn't go away; that is until he tried reflexology, which immediately gave him the relief he craved. Reflexology shows absolutely no preferences when it comes to helping people 'get back onto their feet' and it assists anybody, regardless of their position in life, skin colour, religious conviction or social belief system. All that it requires is complete trust in the process.

> *No amount of pills or potions can heal the pain of non-acceptance!*

02

a complementary art of healing

In this chapter you will learn:
- how reflexology complements medicine
- about helpful lifestyle changes
- about other complementary modalities.

Modern medicine and reflexology

Orthodox medicine is around 300 years old, yet it is still comparatively young in relation to ancient complementary healing methods, such as reflexology, which are centuries old. At one time, massaging the body and feet were an accepted and expected way of life. Today, thanks to medical research, it is so much easier to understand how you and your body tick. This has meant that all forms of natural healing have been able to keep pace with the ongoing changes of human needs, since medical knowledge ensures that incredible advancements can be constantly made. As reflexology constantly strides on, its methods and approaches can be continually adapted and adjusted in such a way that it can meet individual needs. It is now increasingly recognized that the body doesn't just play up for the sake of it. Even Hippocrates, the acknowledged Father of Medicine, stated that the physical body reflects the tremendous impact of emotions, which, in turn, determine the disposition of the mind. He used to assess fluctuations in the body's humours to decide which course of action to take, which is how reflexology works, and why, when used hand in hand with medical and surgical procedures, it helps to accelerate the healing process. Meanwhile the foot massage itself brings much comfort and reassurance to the suffering individual.

Reflexology and modern medicine, when used well together, make a dynamic team.

Teaming up together

Reflexology can't possibly re-align shattered or broken bones but it can reduce swellings and inner tension, as well as ease pain and discomfort to such an extent that it creates the ideal environment for the bones to relax and settle back into their natural position. Modern medicine provides instant solutions to relieve physical pain and mental discomfort, making it an advantageous stepping stone in providing temporary relief allowing emotional and spiritual wounds to be healed, which only you can do. No amount of medication can ever mend a broken heart, yet reflexology can assist you in finding the understanding and solution that lies within you. Thanks to the more holistic approach and open-minded attitude of medical professionals worldwide, reflexology is now frequently prescribed, alongside some of the more conventional treatments, and the results to date have been phenomenal. Combining reflexology and modern medicine has the advantage of integrating ancient wisdom with modern technology. By drawing from either one or both modalities, as their requirements change, individuals are able to take exactly what they need to help themselves and feel so much better about who and what they are.

Comparisons are futile because every body is meant to be unique!

Lifestyle changes

There is now more 'dis-ease' on this planet than ever before and there is no doubt that the state of your body is a direct reflection of the content or discontent of your mind. Health after all is your natural state, whilst 'dis-ease' is an outward display of inner conflict and emotional turmoil, brought to your attention by your current circumstances. It is when you make a huge issue out of something relatively small and insignificant that you are likely to tip the delicate balance between health and 'dis-ease'. It just takes one unhealthy obsession, fed by the incredible temptations of modern-day living, to throw you completely off track with your soul purpose. It's these temptations, more than anything else, that take your focus away from what's important. They deprive you and your soul of the ultimate joy of living a full and rewarding life because your self-esteem and self-worth become sadly impoverished through constant self-criticism. Your health is likely to deteriorate, which leaves you in a poor and unsatisfactory state, regardless of how wealthy you are. Reflexology is the light at the end of the tunnel that can help you to climb out of this dark hole and make worthwhile lifestyle changes from which you can benefit and enjoy superb health.

Overall health means complete harmony within your mind, body and soul.

Other complementary steps

There are many marvellous natural healing modalities, therapies and remedies that can be used alongside or in conjunction with reflexology to enhance the healing process. For instance, the **Alexander Technique** realigns your posture in such a way that your whole body re-energizes itself, the effect of which is magnified through reflexology. Then there's the evocative smells of **aromatherapy**, which, when used to massage feet, add more of a sensual dimension. A popular aromatherapy combination often used at the end of a reflexology session is as follows: *juniper* to clear the mind, *bergamot* to calm the nerves and soothe emotions, *neroli* to boost confidence and *ylang-ylang* to heighten the senses and create a much-needed awareness of innermost needs. Meanwhile, always keep a bottle of '*rescue remedy*' at hand to manage a panic attack or break through persistent thought cycles that erode away at personal well-being.

Colour healing is an integral part of reflexology, either through visualization or through the use of gems and crystals, providing a means of restoring balance whilst re-toning the body and bringing it energetically back into balance (see Appendix I). Rose quartz is the most commonly used gem in reflexology since it encourages self-acceptance. Gently place equal sized stones in the recipient's palms at the beginning of a session, leave them there throughout the massage and then at the end of the session take them and lightly rest them against the recipient's solar plexus reflexes (p. 81) for as long as is needed.

Herbs, well known for their remedial qualities, are also great for complementing reflexology because they too are an incredible means of preserving health, as are **homeopathy** and **naturopathy**, both of which are plant derivatives that alleviate dis-ease naturally, effectively prolonging the empowering effect of reflexology when taken between sessions.

Integrating **music** into a reflexology session is ideal for reorganizing the body molecules in such a way that the whole inner structure realigns itself for overall harmony and greater peace (see Appendix II).

Reiki, of course, is the energetic aspect of reflexology and is used to shift and balance life force energies and to replenish parts that lack vitality, hence the increasing use of the term 'rei-flexology'. Finally, **shiatsu, acupressure** and **acupuncture** clear the natural pathways for energy to access all bodily cells. A combination of reflexology with any of these is really beneficial. However, whether used in conjunction with other therapies, or when used alone, reflexology always ensures that the very best results are attained.

Everybody and everything in your life is essentially neutral. It's the intent that brings out the worst and the best in them!

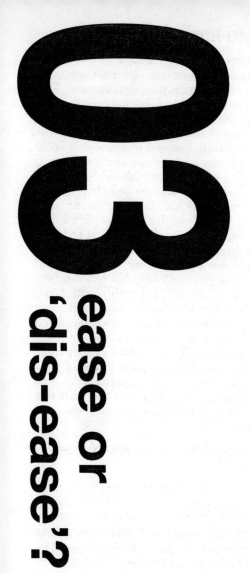

03

ease or 'dis-ease'?

In this chapter you will learn:
- the importance of your approach to life
- what gets in the way of good health
- how to interpret symptoms.

Your approach to life

You have a very special and unique approach to life, which, along with your attitude, determines whether you are emotionally in tune or in conflict with your environment. This, in turn, influences your state of mind and the consequential ease or 'dis-ease' of your body. When you are in good health you are calm, but alert, and up to any challenge, being more receptive to all that comes your way. It's likely that you remain on the look-out for worthwhile opportunities and enthuse about everything that you do whilst showing a greater appreciation of the gift of life. In other words, you 'have a life' and are completely aware of the true art of living. Uneasiness, or 'dis-ease', on the other hand, is the end product of a long list of complaints and ongoing criticism, which highlight your discomfort at trying to live up to the ridiculous expectations of others. Instead of being true to yourself, you and your body become so far removed from your soul's purpose that you can't help but feel intensely frustrated, completely bewildered, incredibly doubtful, extremely unhappy and emotionally lonely. All because you have allowed yourself to conform to limited, often out-dated and unreasonable belief systems, which rob you of your individuality and deny you the many opportunities that came your way. If your memories are filled with the terror of your perceptions they are likely to return and plague you from time to time, making you feel really uneasy about who and what you have become. It's little wonder that there is so much 'dis-ease' and unhappiness in the world today.

Physical symptoms of distress are a sign of inner unhappiness and dissatisfaction.

Re-assessing your life

Whenever resentment builds up inside you, it invariably gets in your way, making you overly anxious and extremely tense. The more you hang onto it, the more discernible it becomes! It hampers you every step of the way, no matter what you try to do to get things going. The physical tension is sometimes too much for your body, especially when it increasingly limits your scope of movement. It can get so bad that you tend to overreact, even though you know that your anger and impatience are completely misplaced, yet you just can't seem to help or control yourself. One of the first things that happens is that it affects your appetite for life, which is why abuse of food has become so widespread. It has become the coping mechanism for many highly evolved souls who feel like 'mis-fits'. Note whether you turn to food for comfort or as a means of concealing your true self. You may be using it to protect yourself against being treated badly. Observe whether you also use alcohol as a means of coping, either to drown your sorrows and give you misplaced bravado, or as a way of celebrating your successes. Determine whether tobacco has become a useful smokescreen, behind which you hide your injured feelings that are far too hurtful to bring out into the open, or whether you use drugs to desensitize yourself from deep inner pain or to remove yourself from having to face and deal with your reality. Everybody abuses something or other, to some extent, at some stage of their life. The good news is that no matter how ill or unhappy you have become, you are always a potentially healthy individual, who, for whatever reason, has temporarily pushed yourself beyond your limits. This, fortunately, forces your to reassess your life and think again, which usually happens when your authenticity is being threatened and you feel completely out of place. When you aren't well, you feel compelled to reconsider your life's circumstances and may even be desperate enough to step into the vast unknown as a means of trying to find something that resonates better with you. This is where reflexology can give you a helping hand.

Symptoms are signs that something is unacceptable to you.

Disturbing your status quo

Whatever disturbs your mind also upsets your body and makes you feel uncomfortable, determining the type of symptom which is then invariably reflected onto your feet. For instance, ulcers indicate that something done or not done is gnawing away and eating at the insides, which shows up in the feet on the related reflex. Meanwhile, the pressure of avoiding emotional conflict is enough to raise blood pressure and cause hypertension, as well as possible tension in the feet. When filled with sadness and remorse, both the body and feet are likely to become heavy and drag themselves through the motions of life. Deep hurt from the past can still overwhelm the heart, making it uneasy and you more susceptible to 'dis-ease'. Also detrimental to personal well-being is an insatiable need for material possessions since it is usually a sign of never feeling 'good enough', which also affects the 'emotional' parts. Then there's that one additional stroke of bad luck or misfortune that paralyses the body with fear, striking it dumb and bringing everything to an abrupt standstill; this is the end result of being overly controlling or from the resentment of others constantly having the upper hand. An ongoing string of soul-destroying disappointments gets to the kidneys and their reflexes, as though they weren't feeling enough of a failure as it was. The point is that illness does not just randomly pick any part of your body in which to create havoc, it's the other way around. When there's chaos in your mind, it is likely to show up in the relevant part of your body and feet, especially when it becomes a problem. It's your body's way of giving you a clue as to what you should do. If you still have no idea what's going on, then just put your feet up and turn to reflexology, because, regardless of your symptoms, it knows how to help you to sort things out in your mind and body.

Symptoms warn you that your body is out of balance.

Reflexology steps in

Whenever there's a crisis, reflexology is delighted to step in. It knows how to deal with uneasiness that comes from disturbing memories and helps you come to terms with the trauma of your past, regardless of how devastating it may have been. For total relief from any form of discomfort, there needs to be a complete shift of mindset and a favourable change of attitude. For instance, if you are constantly irritated by one thing or another and it keeps getting under your skin then you are likely to develop a rash or some other skin disorder. Similarly, if things consistently get up your nose, it's possible that you will be continually bunged up. If life in general has a habit of getting on your nerves then the chances are that you will be exceptionally agitated, highly sensitive or very touchy, all of which are aggravated further by lack of sleep or an unhealthy lifestyle. This can lead to a complete or partial dependency on drugs, food or cigarettes, all of which exacerbate the situation. Your body will show symptoms of ill health until you do something to make things better for yourself and others. This is a good time to invite reflexology into your life; you will be delighted with the new and improved you!

Whatever your mind believes, your body becomes.

Signs that all is not well

Sometimes sickness is the only thing to wake you up to the fact that a massive change is needed in your approach to life. Deep down you know that there is always plenty of room for self-improvement so, by courageously taking steps that are good for you, you will begin to feel so much better about yourself and others, as well as about life in general. Consciously or unconsciously, you have within you the inherent desire to be wholesome, healthy and balanced; you are then able to rely on your internal resourcefulness and inner strength that you have to get through anything and everything. Not only do you discover all that you are really capable of, but you are also likely to rediscover exciting and pleasing aspects of yourself that you may have long since forgotten. Your body is well-equipped to heal itself and stay healthy, if you allow it to. As soon as your body feels better, you feel better. Once you are back on your feet you can step ahead with much greater confidence and with the knowledge of how best to make progress on the next leg of your journey of self-discovery.

Your body talks to you through the ever-changing characteristics of your feet.

The remedy at hand

Fortunately, reflexology is also a great preventative tool. It can pick up and sort out any disturbances in your mind long before they upset your body, which it does by directing vital life forces through energy pathways to immediately dissipate any possible energetic hindrances. It also flushes out mental and emotional congestion, both of which are the physical manifestation of detrimental thought patterns. With less pressure on your mind, your body can relax and function so much better, allowing the surge of new-found energy to infiltrate your whole being. Having said this though, when first giving or receiving reflexology, you may initially feel exhausted and lethargic as old, stale energies, which have been suppressed for some time, begin to surface. However, once your own natural healing resources 'kick in', you will feel so great that there will be no stopping you. You will feel strong enough to overcome any form of adversity, no matter how serious it may seem.

That which you retain inhibits you; that which you release heals you.

04

who benefits from reflexology?

In this chapter you will learn:
- about the benefits of massaging feet
- about the reasons for this
- other fascinating insights.

Anybody and everybody can enjoy and derive enormous benefits from reflexology since it enables each individual to find their own inner peace. The resultant harmony allows their mind and body to function efficiently and effectively which, in turn, raises their spirits. Reflexology is a non-invasive therapy that should be applied sensitively and gently to avoid causing any harm when massaging the feet. Be wary, however, of giving reflexology to anybody with a deep vein thrombosis because, as their muscles relax, the blood clot, usually in their legs, could become dislodged and travel to their brain or heart, with the remote possibility of a stroke or heart attack. Although there has been no report of such an occurrence, it is still advisable to be cautious. Reflexology is particularly beneficial for those who are stuck in a rut, lack direction, feel alone and misunderstood, and for those who constantly question, 'what on earth is the world coming to?' Reflexology can make a world of difference.

The effectiveness of reflexology spans every phase of life.

In pregnancy

Massaging feet during pregnancy (see also pp. 131–5) is enormously beneficial to both the mother-to-be and the unborn baby, particularly when the approach is sensitive and gentle. Together they are able to enjoy this incredible time together, which is, after all, one of the most remarkable and best periods in a woman's life. When the mother-to-be's body is relaxed, there is a constant flow of natural life force energies, which creates an inner peace and a calm environment providing ample space for the unborn baby to grow and develop, thereby reducing the risk of complications. Furthermore, with a livelier blood circulation, both mother and baby are kept well nourished, which bodes well for a much stronger bond of trust and pure love after the birth.

Mothers-to-be and their unborn children thrive on reflexology.

Babies and children

Babies and children are energetically, and often painfully, aware of their parent's thoughts and feelings, so much so that their well-being is intrinsically linked. This is why, whenever a child is sick, the parent, especially the mum, should be treated as well. Children mirror what's really going on at home, long before their parents are even aware that there could be a problem. Fortunately, youngsters generally love to have their feet massaged and usually respond particularly well, especially those who tend to be ultra-sensitive. Reflexology is also great for hyperactive children, who have such a hard time trying to conform. With greater inner calm, youngsters can relate so much better to themselves and others. In this way, reflexology can help each child acknowledge their true spirit so that they can grow up to be the individual that they are really meant to be.

Children reflect their parents; as their parents get better, the children get better.

Teenagers

Adolescents are well tuned into universal energies, but they are often reluctant to admit to it for fear of not fitting in. However, whether they like it or not, they do tend to respond incredibly well to having their feet massaged, especially when it comes to balancing their mind, body and spirit at the onset of puberty. It will also assist them with the ongoing distribution of hormones, and naturally helps them to feel much more comfortable about being themselves. Reflexology also encourages them to have more trusting and honest relationships, so that, with greater self-assurance, they can easily step into adulthood with improved tolerance and more poise.

Teenagers can actually feel good about being so different.

Adults

Adulthood is the time when individuals can really get to know what they are made of and realize what it is that makes them tick. The sooner they understand that the only thing getting in their way is themselves, the sooner they get better at being themselves! Reflexology helps them to realize that it's okay to be 'out of the ordinary' and extra-ordinary. As they let go of self-induced pressures, there are less wrinkles of concern and anxiety. Also, as hefty burdens and weighty issues are lifted from their minds, their bodies stop sagging in despair. Massaging the feet encourages adults to become more lenient with themselves, whilst having greater tolerance for others. It also minimizes the damaging effect of distress, fear and worry through the restoration of their faith in life's processes. As adults become more relaxed, there is not such an intense need to be so much in control.

Reflexology puts us in a much happier and healthier frame of mind and body.

Seniors

Reflexology is a wonderful gift to oneself when growing older. It comes with numerous advantages, such as keeping the mind, body and soul agile and alert, whilst injecting the whole being with renewed enthusiasm for life. As seniors become fitter, they rediscover their true meaning and purpose of being here, whilst massaging their feet also helps them to improve their concentration, so that they can really focus on the more worthwhile aspects of their life. At the same time, it ensures a quicker turnover of tired worn-out cells so that they can be frequently replenished with new, vibrant and healthy cells.

Seniors can spring back into action and make the most of the rest of their lives.

Distressed souls

Whenever feeling unwell, upset or confused, having your feet massaged can provide instant relief; it is the very best thing that you can do for yourself and others. It meets your desperate need to be touched and cared for, whilst, at the same time, relieving you of your aches and pains. You soon become less vulnerable and don't feel so defenceless, with your sense of hopelessness soon dissipating. Destructive emotions and devastating thoughts that used to get in your way become things of the past, enabling new, healthy and rejuvenated energies to step in and take their place. By having your feet massaged, you receive all the reassurance you need: your mind can clear, your body can realign itself and your soul can feel loved and worthwhile.

Reflexology makes you feel so much better about being you.

The family unit

Even if you are the only member in your family to receive reflexology, everybody at home benefits, because you become such a pleasure to live with! When the whole family enjoys a foot massage, or, better still, massage each other's feet, the outcome is incredible. The gap between generations is bridged, with greater respect and love being shown to one another. Everybody accepts everybody else for who and what they are. Each individual can then feel really happy that they belong to such an understanding family unit.

You feel so much better with peace of mind, a relaxed body and a contented soul.

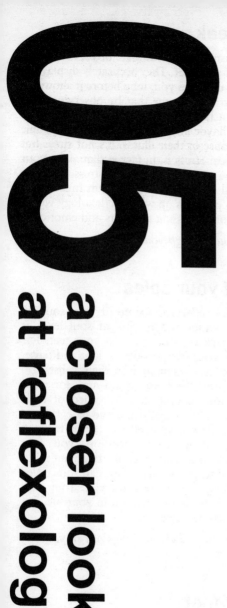

05

a closer look at reflexology

In this chapter you will learn:
- the language of the feet
- how reflexology works
- about the condition of your feet.

Let your feet speak

Just as symptoms of 'dis-ease' reflect your state of your mind, so too do the characteristics of your feet. They accurately display the root cause of anything that unsettles you, long before it shows up as a disorder in your body. This means that by observing your feet, potential problems can be seen and dealt with before they disrupt your life and cause havoc in your body. Yet, many people still see stress as the root cause of their illness. It's not stress but distress that upsets your body. Stress is, in fact, essential for your well-being since it keeps you upright and alert. Distress, however can cause your body to fall apart and stops it from functioning well. Your feet are quick to pick this up whilst reflexology works immediately by getting rid of distressing thoughts and emotions.

Your body speaks to you through your feet!

The condition of your soles

The condition of your soles reflects the state of your soul; so much so that whenever anything upsets you, at soul level, it immediately shows up as lack of composure in your feet. For instance, if you feel uneasy, your feet become uptight and tense. Similarly, lack of energy causes them to lose their substance, making it really difficult for them to 'stand up' for you. Whenever you feel off colour your feet are drained of their vibrancy, making them look rather insignificant and pale. If, over a period of time, you have allowed yourself to become trapped in a compromising or disadvantageous position, you may temporarily 'disable' yourself, as a result of contorting your mind to such an extent that you distort your feet. This can sometimes be so severe that they no longer work well for you. Your feet, through their condition, reflect what's going on in your life and how you really feel at a much deeper level.

Reflexology knows how to straighten things out in your mind, body and feet.

Literally 'at your feet'

There are many expressions with 'foot' or 'feet' in them, which are frequently used to symbolically describe your standing and situation in life. Whenever in a fortunate position, you may be said to have 'landed on your feet', and when you are presented with a new situation, you may be trying to 'find your feet'. By 'putting your best foot forward' you can make a good impression, whilst every time you 'put your foot down', it could imply that you are taking a firm stand and possibly being rather obstinate! Then there's the embarrassment of 'opening your mouth' and 'putting your foot in it', or the pain of being 'trampled under foot' when your ideas are oppressed or treated with contempt. This is a good time to 'be on good footing' with your friends and acquaintances. Your feet provide fascinating insight into who and what you are and, in so doing, provide a basic understanding of your unique requirements. Reflexology tends to bring out, first the worst, then the best in you so that you can really get ahead in life.

Your feet reveal the story of your life.

Get ahead through your feet

Feet provide you with a solid foundation and, at the same time, give you the flexibility to move ahead and make progress. They are your roots and, as such, afford you the security you crave, as well as the stability you need to adjust to all the unexpected ups and downs that you encounter. From time to time, fear, uncertainty and anxiety step in and invariably get in your way. As soon as you experience self-doubt because you are so 'unsure of your footing', your feet become less flexible. This makes your journey more arduous and heavy-going and you are then more likely to 'trip over your own two feet'. Once you feel secure, content and happy about 'standing on your own two feet', you soon find it much easier to get 'a foot in the door' and 'step ahead' with a 'spring in your step'. You are more able to adjust to the unexpected twists and turns of life, making you realize that life is an exciting adventure of your mind and that it can take you wherever you wish to go!

Everybody is headed for an unknown destination.

How reflexology works

The 'extra-ordinary' and often miraculous way in which reflexology rejuvenates, refreshes and restores cannot be fully explained, since any form of healing ultimately comes from the universe. To get an idea of what happens, it helps first to visualize the impact of distress on your mind, body and soul, since fear, anxiety and distrust can have a devastating effect on your insides, physically, mentally, emotionally and spiritually. Your body instinctively defends itself from possible attack by preparing your cells, which then makes you uneasy, further tensing your body and feet and increasing the likelihood of adverse reactions as your muscles contract and clamp mercilessly down on your body. Your capacity to function is greatly reduced and your feet, detecting this insecurity and uncertainty, become increasingly rigid. With reduced mobility, you are held back, depriving your cells of their full blood quota, which in turn starves your whole body of its vital life force energies. As you become drained of your inner strength and resourcefulness, your feet weaken and can barely hold themselves upright. Everything comes to a virtual standstill, denying you the opportunity to grow and develop. Instead potentially dangerous substances, such as toxic thoughts and noxious emotions, become trapped inside you. There is further chaos as you feel more and more overwhelmed and burdened making your feet swell and possibly harden as a cover-up or to conceal your vulnerability. This is a good time to help your body out through your feet.

Reflexology works by healing your mind, body and soul at a sub-conscious level. It avoids causing you any further emotional disstress by sunconsciously dealing with outstanding traumatic memories at a much deeper level. The massage itself dissipates tension by coaxing your uptight muscles to release their intense grip so that you can let go of potentially harmful substances which immediately takes weight off your mind, calms you inwardly and lifts your spirit. With less pressure, your frazzled nerves are soothed and can start functioning as they should. Meanwhile, distraught emotions are calmed, creating a far more peaceful internal environment, which is absolutely necessary for deep healing to take place.

Sluggish, hypo-active glands or organs are stimulated and brought back to life through reflexology, whilst any over-excited, hyperactive parts are calmed down; either way your glands and organs can return to functioning far more efficiently and effectively. With increased elasticity throughout your whole body, you become much more flexible and mobile which, in turn, boosts your blood flow, so much so, that all your cells are generously replenished and well-nurtured. They then have plenty of energy with which to rejuvenate themselves, whilst, at the same time, restoring you.

With the efficient functioning of your whole being, your good health is ensured.

From the inside out

Reflexology soothes from the inside out and, as such, is an extremely impressive antidote to distress. Whilst having your feet massaged, you may drift into the most exquisite and deeply relaxing alpha state of consciousness, which is the tranquillity enjoyed between wakefulness and sleep. If your mind, body and soul take full advantage of this autonomy, they can totally regroup and fully recuperate their energies. Your body is then able to rejuvenate itself without any interference. It does this by constantly forming billions of new cells to keep you well up-dated and in excellent working condition. When relaxed, you are naturally able to re-energize yourself by absorbing universal energy from two main sources, the sun and the earth. The hairs on your head and body soak up the vibrant, light, positive male energies of the sun, whilst the soles of your feet suck up the solid, dark, mysterious female energies from the earth; reflexology increases this receptiveness. As various organs and glands take on this vibrancy, their energy rebounds back to the surface, which is how you know what's going on inside your body, through the ever-changing characteristics of your body and your feet.

Knowledge is attained through positive and negative actions and reactions, with health being the neutral position of life.

A powerful relaxation technique

All perceived adversities, no matter how large or small, can either be a destructive force or used to your advantage. It's your choice. You can either be the victim or you can grab the opportunity with both hands and become more of yourself, with reflexology helping you to overcome any perceived adversity. The relief of letting go is so great that you instinctively know how to get back on track, making it so much easier to stay in touch with your soul mission. As soon as you allow your mind to accept and express your individuality, whilst doing something really worthwhile with your talents, you become filled with love for yourself and others. Reflexology encourages you to constantly improve on yourself and, in so doing, enjoy an enhanced quality of life. As a powerful relaxation technique its advantages are enormous, particularly in this frenetic age of relentless speed and endless deadlines. Maybe if 'dead lines' were called 'live lines' every body would feel so much better!

For healing to occur it's important to go with, not against, the manifestation of illness and 'dis-ease'.

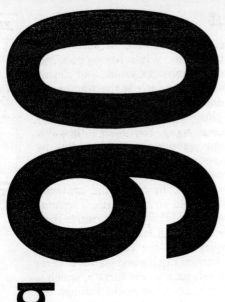

06

body reflections

In this chapter you will learn:
- how your body is depicted onto your feet
- what to look for
- the importance of both sides.

Ongoing knowledge

Reflexology is based on knowledge that has been handed down from generation to generation for thousands of years. The information has been relayed so many times, over such a huge expanse of time, that it's inevitable that the interpretation of reflexes do vary slightly, according to each individual's understanding. The result is a fair assortment of foot charts, which, although basically the same, have been adjusted in some instances. The reflexes most affected by these discrepancies are the spine, ears, eyes, heart, breasts and knees.

Also with many of the organs, glands and parts overlapping in the body, it means that several reflexes can be present in one specific part of the foot. For instance, your nerves, blood and lymph vessels infiltrate your whole body, whilst your bones and muscles form your basic infrastructure, so these reflexes naturally abound throughout every part of both feet. Furthermore, there is more than one way to access a reflex, either via the primary reflex, which gives you direct access, or via the secondary or indirect reflex, which approaches the area from behind, usually on the opposite side of the foot. For example, breasts are reflected directly onto the balls of both feet, but can still be accessed via their secondary or indirect reflexes, on the tops of the feet (figure 1).

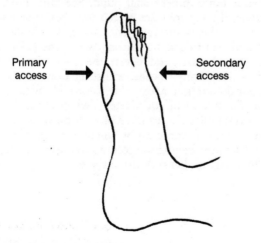

Primary
access

Secondary
access

figure 1 primary and secondary breast reflexes

Picture your body on your feet

You can see how perfectly all your body parts are reflected onto your feet by simply visualizing the insides of your body in miniature on your own feet or, better still, on somebody else's feet (see figure 2, pp. 29–30) with their feet in front of you. When your two feet are together, they represent your whole body, with your front mirrored onto your soles and your back depicted on top. The right side of your body is reflected onto your right foot, whilst your left foot corresponds with the left side of your body. The accuracy of this is so great that, wherever a part of your body is missing or removed, there is a corresponding gap or hollow on the matching part of the foot. Conversely any extra bones and organs will soon show up in their related areas, as their energies rebound back to the surface. Deep inner scar tissue can be felt as hardness, whilst bones that are crushed have a shattered, splintered or gritty feel to their reflexes. It helps enormously to visualize the various parts of the body on the feet when doing reflexology.

Sit in front of a mirror, with your legs stretched out in front of you and your soles placed side by side, or alternatively invite somebody else to do the same. Then visualize the body parts on a substantially smaller scale, as follows. Your face is represented on your cushioned toe pads, with each toe revealing different aspects of your multi-dimensional mind. See how, more often than not, when the big toes are placed together, they resemble the shape of your head and face. Moving down the feet, your toe necks mirror your neck and throat, whilst the balls of your feet reflect your breasts and chest; the solidarity of which corresponds to your bony ribcage, whilst the dome at their base looks like your diaphragm. Meanwhile your abdominal cavity is linked to the fleshy part of your insteps, whereas the denseness of your heels resembles the firmness of your bony pelvis. It's all there, on full view, for you to know where to place your fingers and thumbs when massaging the feet, as well as to get a feel of what is really going on beneath the surface.

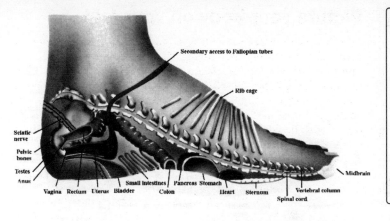

Secondary access to Fallopian tubes

Rib cage

Sciatic nerve

Pelvic bones

Testes

Anus

Vagina Rectum Uterus Bladder Small intestines Colon Pancreas Stomach Heart Sternum Spinal cord Vertebral column Midbrain

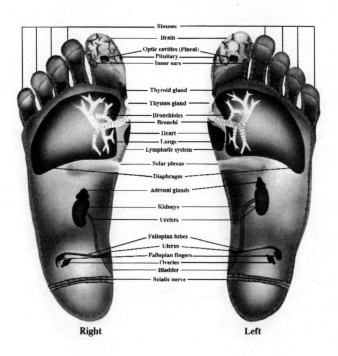

Sinuses
Brain
Optic cavities (Pineal)
Pituitary
Inner ears
Thyroid gland
Thymus gland
Bronchioles
Bronchi
Heart
Lungs
Lymphatic system
Solar plexus
Diaphragm
Adrenal glands
Kidneys
Ureters
Fallopian tubes
Uterus
Fallopian fingers
Overies
Bladder
Sciatic nerve

Right   Left

figure 2 reflection of bodily parts in miniature on the feet

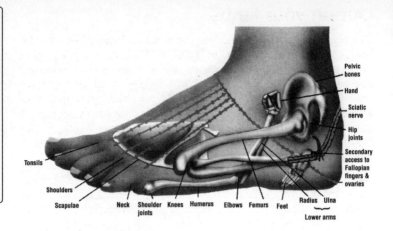

Pelvic bones

Hand

Sciatic nerve

Hip joints

Secondary access to Fallopian fingers & ovaries

Tonsils

Shoulders

Scapulae

Neck

Shoulder joints

Knees

Humerus

Elbows

Femurs

Feet

Radius

Ulna

Lower arms

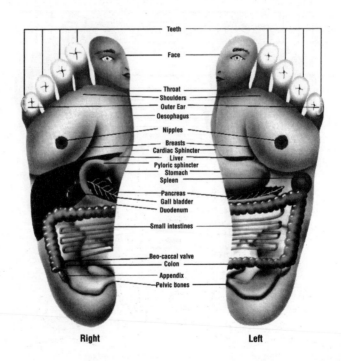

Teeth

Face

Throat

Shoulders

Outer Ear

Oesophagus

Nipples

Breasts

Cardiac Sphincter

Liver

Pyloric sphincter

Stomach

Spleen

Pancreas

Gall bladder

Duodenum

Small intestines

Beo-caccal valve

Colon

Appendix

Pelvic bones

Right

Left

Out on your limbs

The upper surfaces of your feet are solid and firm, just like the back of your body, which they accurately reflect. They may also display marks and impressions from your past, reflecting unpleasant situations that you 'put behind you' or went on 'behind your back' or to reveal difficult memories that you shoved 'into the background', along with those who you 'turned your back on'. A whole range of 'back' sayings highlight the basis of back problems, of which there is an alarming epidemic worldwide.

Just beneath your little toes are prominent bones that reflect your upper arm sockets, whilst halfway down the outer edges are bony protrusions, which correspond to your elbows. From these mounds take a 45 degree line to your outer ankle bones, where the fist-like mounds mirror your hands. The outlines of your outer ankle bones mimic the edges of your hip bones, from which your leg reflexes extend as shown below (figure 3).

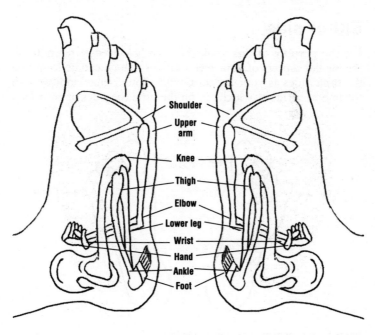

figure 3 back and limb reflexes on the outer edges of both feet

Your lower limbs are also reflected onto the soles of both feet; in the same seated position, with your knees bent up against the body (figure 4).

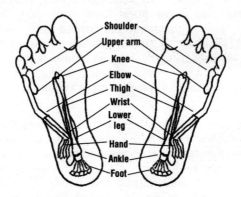

figure 4 limb reflexes on the soles of both feet

Either side

For the purpose of this book the term 'inner edge' refers to all the medial aspects of your feet and toes, which can be found on the same sides as your big toes, whilst 'outer edge' indicates all the lateral surfaces, which are on the little toe sides of your feet.

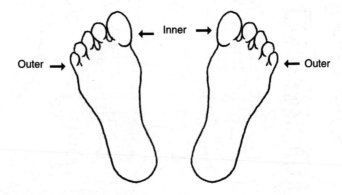

figure 5 inner and outer aspects of the feet

Feet are perfect microcosms of your mind, body and soul.

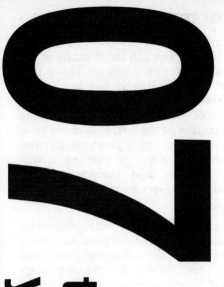

07

the power of your touch

In this chapter you will learn:
- the way to touch
- how best to embrace feet
- the most effective ways to get results.

The importance of touch

Your personal touch is the most important aspect of reflexology and your touch is unique. Nobody else can touch others in the same way that you do, no matter how hard they try. This is why you should never try to emulate anybody else. Just be yourself. Others quickly pick up on how you feel, the moment you touch them, so always be conscious of your feelings before massaging feet. Any form of caress, especially of the feet, evokes emotion, either consciously or subconsciously, which is why aggressive, threatening actions make the body recoil or lash out in self-defence whereas acts of kindness and acceptance boost confidence and create a trusting environment that makes life seem so much more manageable.

When giving reflexology, make sure that you touch others with supreme sensitivity, the purest of intent and complete acceptance of who and what they are. Then use the massage to loosen and break down the fixation with time, so that they can now let go of inhibiting and intimidating belief systems, as well as dreadful memories that are well past their sell-by date. The therapeutic movements of your touch can and do make a world of difference.

Making contact

Until recently the reflexology technique concentrated mainly on the all-important physical and mechanical aspects of being human. As times have changed, it has now expanded to embrace all modern needs, making it one of the most all-encompassing therapies available. As you touch the recipient's feet, you will soon know how to tune into their energies and will innately be aware of the type of touch that they need to feel better, whether it should be firm, medium or light. A general rule of thumb is that those who have a more physical approach to life tend to prefer a more definite, harder massage (although, at times, they benefit greatly from the gentler touch), whilst the more emotional, spiritually aware souls generally favour a softer, non-physical massage, yet they often need to be grounded with a slightly firmer touch. The need to be touched and nurtured increases during times of illness, distress or insecurity, with the therapeutic touch being exceptionally well received since it eases distress, pacifies emotions, reassures the soul, induces confidence, creates trust and increases acceptance of oneself and others.

Healing through your hands

When giving reflexology, try using all your fingers and both thumbs because each digit has its own unique energy, which alters the vibration and eventual effect of your touch. It also introduces a far greater range of healing possibilities and enhances the overall effect of the massage. Your thumbs help the recipient to trust again and create a much-needed balance between their intellect and intuition. Your second fingers allow them to feel again, so that they can reconnect with their innermost emotions and just be themselves. Then your middle fingers activate their mind so that they know exactly what to do with all those amazing ideas, making them more aware of their capabilities, whilst your ring fingers assist them in relating to their new concepts, giving them the courage to communicate and share these and, in so doing, discover more about themselves. As for your powerful little fingers, don't be deceived by their size! They encourage the recipient to expand beyond tried and tested boundaries so that they become more of themselves, knowing that they are unique and have come to make a difference. All in all, your digits make an amazing team that help bring out the very best in others.

For the best results

Whether you give reflexology to ease specific symptoms or for the maintenance of health, to derive the best possible results, massage every single reflex thoroughly, with a combination of all four movements (pp. 136–40), concentrating on the brain (p. 42), spinal (p. 52), solar plexus (p. 81) and endocrine gland (p. 178) reflexes. It may initially take you an hour and a half to two hours to complete a full treatment but, with confidence and practice, this can be reduced to around an hour. Also spend extra time on congested, swollen areas or parts that lack energy and vibrancy. These can be easily felt on the feet: fear, anxiety or vulnerability cause a resistance or hardness; exhaustion or a need for some serious attention causes a 'sucking' sensation; whilst a reflex that is drained of its energy often feels dull, flat or unresponsive. On all these areas, lightly rest any digit and gently but firmly 'pump' the reflex until a gush of energy is felt. Alternatively, use the rotation technique (p. 137) to reawaken and stimulate the reflex. You will also soon be able to detect sluggish, hypo-active, unresponsive areas that need re-activating, as well as hyperactive or tense areas that need pacifying. Even if you can't feel anything, don't worry; the body knows what to do, thanks to the impetus that you give it through the feet.

The best way of doing anything has never been found.

Give credit where it's due

Whenever you trust your intuition to guide you, you are likely to be absolutely amazed at the incredible results as they occur before your very eyes! Within minutes there can be such great shifts in energy that, by the end of one session, the benefits are really obvious. Resist the temptation, however, to take credit for these phenomenal occurrences, since you are merely the conduit. Just remember that the recipient, in deciding to get better, has drawn on the Universal source to help themselves to better health. When you don't take the credit for the healing, you won't lose confidence if, from time to time, the recipient doesn't wish to improve.

Sometimes being ill and helpless serves them more because of all the sympathy and attention they receive, which either slows down or blocks the healing process. Others prefer to remain incapacitated because they feel incapable of meeting outrageous expectations. This is why it is so important never to try to impose your will upon another soul. You would obviously love to see them get better, but sometimes they have to go through whatever it is that they need to experience to get to where they are going. No matter how painful or long-winded it may seem to you, it serves them at this stage of their life. The best you can do is to keep offering them the opportunity to get better through reflexology.

Many see themselves as the victims of change and circumstances, instead of seeing the opportunity for growth and development.

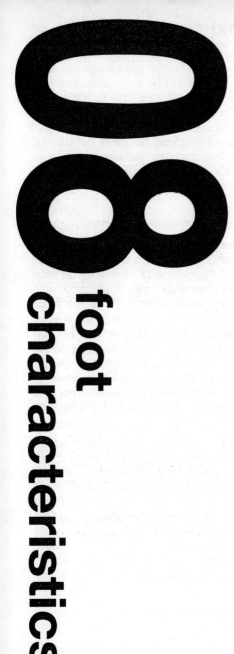

08
foot characteristics

In this chapter you will learn:
- about the healing qualities of colour
- what's left and what's right
- how to improve your angle on life.

Take a closer look!

When doing reflexology, you have the ideal opportunity to have a really good look at the feet and observe any changes in their characteristics. The shifts can be really noticeable and can happen surprisingly quickly. They will help you to have a far better idea of where the recipient is coming from, as well as all that they have been through, on their sometimes treacherous journey through life. Those who survive the most devastating circumstances and come out a stronger person inspire others to do the same and are often the best at extending their hand in helping others to heal themselves since they have been through so much themselves.

As far as a person falls is as high as they can rise.

In their natural state, your feet are vibrant and pliant, making it so much easier for them to adapt and fit into the ever-changing circumstances of your life and they are quick to pick up on your feelings. For instance, if you are anxious upset or alarmed, they can be extremely unforgiving which makes them far more susceptible to injury and 'dis-ease'. It's when you allow your past and all those negative memories to get in your way that you experience endless frustrations. As soon as the going gets tough, the skin on your feet hardens and thickens, sometimes in specific positions, known as calluses or corns, to highlight areas of extreme vulnerability, whilst, at the same time, protecting you and helping you conceal your true feelings or, alternatively, to hide your inadequacies.

Your feet become flaccid when you give in too easily under pressure or when you lack the inner strength and substance to keep going; whereas they toughen up at times when you are having to be extra resourceful to get through a difficult patch. If you are continually being 'rubbed up the wrong way', your skin becomes shiny, whereas it flakes in a desperate attempt to get rid of all those pesky irritabilities that keep 'getting under your skin' or because you have a 'flaky' approach to life. Whenever you undergo a complete change of mind or experience a total transition, your skin is likely to peel away as the old makes way for the new.

Be daring and think of what to change.

Colour

Your feet are naturally flesh-coloured to comfortably blend in with the changing hues that colour your journey through life. Several different colours can come to the surface at any one time and can perpetually change as your overriding moods and uppermost emotions fluctuate from one extreme to the other, sometimes in a matter of seconds. There are a few significant colours that appear on the feet: *white* is indicative of being absolutely drained, tired and exhausted or a sign of divine guidance and enlightenment; *black* or *blue* indicates being momentarily in the dark and needing an expressive outlet, or alternatively from being really hurt and emotionally battered, with the depth of colour indicating the severity of injured feelings; tinges of *green* come from extreme envy or a profound need to just be; *yellow* indicates exceptional annoyance or a jaundiced view of life at the one extreme, whilst being overly conscientious at the other; *orange*, being a mixture of red and yellow, often reveals mixed emotions, generally veering more towards being really fed up and confused; *red* is generally a sign of heated emotions, intense rage, extreme frustration or total embarrassment (otherwise it is surfacing passion); *brown* could be due to being 'browned off' or needing to feel more grounded and in touch with nature (or the feet are just dirty!).

Colour the world with your own brand of ingenuity.

Left and right

The energies that you absorb from the sun and the earth are channelled through your whole body, giving you a balanced view of life. Whilst you have two eyes, two ears, two arms, two legs and two feet, it is your head, neck and body that brings everything together. You will always be connected to your past through your back and the right side of your body, whilst being able to reach out to your future through the front and left side of your body; with your central core keeping you well in the present. As you stride ahead, one foot in front of the other, you gain far greater understanding of yourself and others by coming from both sides. So take a look at your feet to see how your right foot reflects the right side of your body and leans more heavily towards your past, being more influenced by the men in your life, as well as those who are older than you. Then glance at your left foot, which represents the left side of your body and draws on the dark, mysterious energies of the earth, being more affected by the women in your life or those who are younger than you. Each cell balances this out by containing both male and female energies, with the positive and negative input coming from your dominant thoughts, uppermost feelings, past actions and immediate reactions. It really does depend on whether you favour one side more than the other because this influences the relationship between your two feet.

Whatever is on the one side always affects the other.

Angle

The angle of your feet signifies your perceived position and bearing in life, which varies depending on whether you are walking, standing, sitting or lying. These differing angles have much to say about your inclination to get on with life or your tendency to hold yourself back. When walking, your feet point in the direction in which you are headed. If your feet are parallel, then you are on track with your soul intentions, but, if they are too open you are being far too accommodating and need to stop trying to please others all the time. Being pigeon-toed shows a lack of confidence or a subconscious need to withdraw and go within, possibly to do some soul-searching. Then there's the space between your feet when you stand which reveals how open you are to what's going on, as well as the scope of your interest. When your feet 'stand to attention' you are likely to be on your best behaviour or very focused or shut off for a while. Meanwhile when you are seated your toes generally point in the direction of your greatest interest, unless you are putting on an act! Whilst lying on your back, your feet should be upright but relaxed: if they pull over to the right, a past concern may be holding you back or your may think back a lot; whereas if they go to the left, then you are more likely to be ahead of yourself with constant forward planning. Feet may keep changing their position throughout a reflexology session, so take note of this, especially when the recipient jerks, snores or pulls a face; it will give you an idea of where their mind is and what may be going on at a sub-conscious level.

The characteristics of your feet reveal the true story of your life.

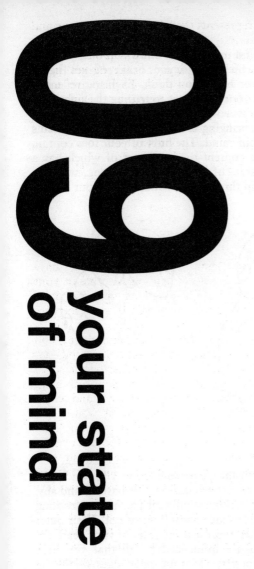

09

your state of mind

In this chapter you will learn:
- about your toes
- about the workings of your mind
- what's at the back of your mind.

Brain reflexes

Whatever is on your mind immediately shows up on your feet, especially in your toes, which contain your brain reflexes (figure 6), revealing how well or badly you think. Each toe reflects a part of your head, with your right toes mirroring the right side, drawing attention to how you used to think, whilst your left toes reflect the left side, bringing to the fore the effect of what's currently going on in your mind. The bulk of your toes contain your brain reflexes, the content or discontent of which has a direct impact on your state of health and well-being, with the overall effect showing up through the condition of your feet.

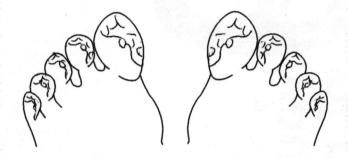

figure 6 brain reflexes on all toes

Toe pads

Your toe pads mirror your face, exposing the way in which you 'face life', whether you are confrontational or bashful and shy. They also mirror what you think of all that you are confronting and whether you are able to face life full on or not. Their outer edges, on the little toe side, represent the sides of your head, the characteristics of which are influenced by all that you hear within your family and society, whilst the inner edges, on the big toe side, represent the inside of your head, where everything comes together to form your core beliefs.

key   T = thoughts
      F = feelings
      D = doing, actions and reactions
      C = communications and relationships
      S = basic security

figure 7 specific toe meanings

Toe by toe

Each set of your toes reflects a different aspect of your multi-dimensional mind and of your thinking process. Your 'intellectual' *big* toes resonate to your innermost beliefs, as well as to your intuitive and spiritual choices; your 'emotional' *second* toes are full of what you think and feel about yourself and others. Your 'energetic' *third* toes have a host of bright ideas of what you should or should not be doing with your life; whilst your 'chatty' *fourth* toes contain views regarding your relationships and also your ability to communicate; leaving your *little* 'family' toes disclose how secure you feel according to your perceived status in life.

The toes divide into six horizontal sections and a closer look at each section reveals a more detailed picture of your mental and intellectual state.

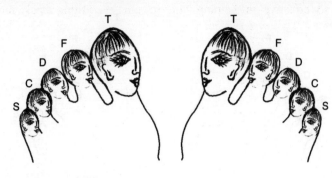

key   big toes = thinking
second toes = feeling
third toes = doing
fourth toes = communications
fifth toes = security

figure 8 facial reflexes and their meanings

Brain, hair and sinuses

Along the tops of all toes are your brain, hair and sinuses reflexes, revealing your capacity to 'think off the top of your head'. It's your brain that helps you to reason, whilst your sinuses give you the space in which to think and your hair acts as your antennae, showing the power of your mind. Concentrate on these reflexes to soothe extreme sensitivity, to ease intense irritability and to increase your level of tolerance, especially when suffering from *sinus congestion, allergies* or fits of rage. Spend extra time on these parts for *baldness*, to mentally stop 'pulling your hair out' and to be free of the intellectual strain of doubt and uncertainty. These reflexes should also be massaged for *depression* so that greater light can be thrown on darker memories; for *dizziness* and vertigo to prevent upsetting thoughts from going round and round in your head; for *fainting* so that you know that you can cope, even when everything else is collapsing around you; for *headaches*, with the understanding that progress is still possible as things come to a head; for *insomnia* to put your mind at rest so that your body and soul can follow suit; and also for *nervousness* to restore your faith in your own capabilities. These top sections on your toes are energetically linked to your big toes, thumbs, tips of your fingers, hands and feet, as well as to your nervous, endocrine and sensory systems. This is why massaging them is so effective in helping you to put everything back into perspective.

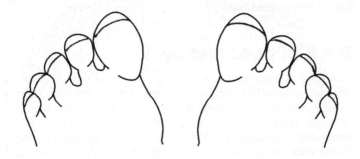

figure 9 brain, hair and sinus reflexes

Forehead and midbrain

Stretched along the next strips (figure 10), which are a continuation of the previous section, are your forehead and midbrain reflexes that display the nature of your thoughts, as well as the impression you gain whenever you have the courage to express your own ideas. Favourable reactions soothe and relax your brow, whilst others 'frowning' on your ideas, causes your temple to wrinkle with concern, making your forehead furrowed and divided. Pay extra additional attention to these strips for *Bell's palsy*, for the courage to face the world as a unique individual and for a *brain tumour* to replace toxic thoughts with exciting new concepts. These reflexes are energetically linked to your toe necks, shoulders, wrists and

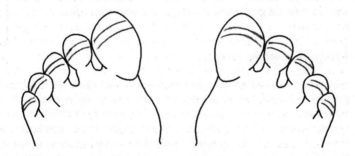

figure 10 forehead reflexes

ankles. They rely on your lymphatic system to keep your body open through the constant clearance of impurities so that you can openly express yourself. Massaging these strips clears the way for you to be yourself.

Back of head and neck

The back of your head and neck are reflected onto the tops of all your toes to illustrate all that goes on 'at the back of your mind', whereas your toenails represent your skull to show, through their characteristics, how well you care for and safeguard your thoughts. Your nails change their appearance by *thickening,* when you believe that your ideas need extra protection against criticism or mockery or whenever you try desperately to cling onto out-dated thoughts and self-imposed systems; they become *vertically ridged* in areas that need to be guarded particularly well; and develop *horizontal ridges* at times of increased vulnerability; or they *lift* or *fall off* as a subconscious means of bringing radical thoughts or innermost fears 'out into the open'. Individuals tend to tear at their toe nails when, metaphysically, they are 'tearing their hair out' and have no idea of what else to do; whilst others resort to biting their toe nails when extremely anxious about moving ahead because of extreme uncertainty.

Another way in which ideas and beliefs are subconsciously protected from attack is through corns. If they are above the toe pads they stop others from 'stamping out ideas', whilst those that are a little lower down, above the toe necks, are to avoid 'getting it in the neck'. Corns on the outer edges are from constantly 'turning a deaf ear'. Reflexology gives you the confidence to believe in yourself and your great thoughts, so that you no longer need to shield or cover them up.

Belief systems

Social constraints and limited belief systems are responsible for putting a huge amount of pressure on your mind, which limits your capacity to think and prevents you from fully utilizing your brain. Whenever you worry about what others may think or not think, or whenever you are fearful of the social consequences of what may happen should you do or not do something, you retreat into conforming to unreasonable belief systems, whether you like them or not. Your muscles instantly contract, substantially reducing the size of your cranium, which puts even more pressure on your brain and deprives your brain cells of their essential life forces. This, in turn, denies them the opportunity to function to their greatest capacity. Whenever you are too terrified to speak up your truth, you are likely to experience a loss of concentration, extreme irritability, great impatience, constant headaches, incessant migraine, increasing baldness, fits of frustration, distorted senses or exaggerated perceptions, which are all signs of deep discontent. Reflexology frees you from inhibiting belief systems and encourages you to utilize your brain cells fully so that you can achieve all that you came to do, regardless of what others may think or say. After all, they are only expressing their own frustration and it is unlikely that they are being true to themselves anyway.

Your state of mind

The 'stature' of your toes reveals your state of mind and also shows your degree of confidence in standing up for yourself and facing the world as 'you'. In their natural state, they hold themselves upright, yet are pliant, firm and flexible. However, your toes immediately become rigid when set beliefs, an unbending attitude or an obdurate approach to life take over, made worse by increasing uncertainty and insecurity. They may stiffen with strong determination. They may even lean forwards, over your soles, whenever you frantically try to put your point of view across, or whenever you 'stick your neck out' or at times when you are 'in another's face'; or they may 'bow' either from subservience or from going head first into life.

Your toes are likely to pull themselves back, away from your soles, when you withdraw or hold back your own ideas, often as a way of avoiding confrontation or occasionally to draw on previous knowledge. Meanwhile they slant to the right for ancient wisdom or when preoccupied with the past or they lean over to the left when drawn to the future or because you are a visionary. Reflexology encourages you to face the world with your own unique and unusual concepts, reminding you that you came into this world to make a big difference.

10

toe characteristics

In this chapter you will learn:
- how you shape your mind
- about the space in which you think
- the impact of your thoughts.

Shape

The shape of your toes reveals how your ideas take shape, which, in turn, influences the shape of things to come. They change their shape whenever you think in a particular way or whenever you have a complete change of mind and, in so doing, have much to say about how you form your opinions. For instance, they become *misshapen* when you contort your mind and try to fit into belief patterns that aren't yours; they appear *boxed* from having to contain all those amazing ideas, which you keep a firm lid on for fear of the dreadful consequences; they become *pointed* when you 'go straight to the point' often with sharp, witty or, sometimes, hurtful comments; they look *squashed* when you quell your notions, even before they have had a chance to take shape; they become *dented* from you constantly knocking your ideas because you believe that they are inadequate or ridiculous. Reflexology helps you to think better of yourself and others so that you can mould a far better reality for yourself and see your life take shape the way you would like it to.

Size

Meanwhile, the size of your toes shows how well you size up yourself and others, based on your belief systems and experiences. This then affects your capacity to think. *Larger* toes provide more space in which to play around with ideas, although it could also mean that you are prone to procrastination! *Smaller* toes may indicate that you are a quick thinker but don't always take the time to think things through. Toes *shrink* when you are denied the opportunity to think for yourself or if you have a deep fear of what others may think. Alternatively they expand and become *overly large* when you are bursting with brilliant notions that have no perceivable outlet; it may also imply that you are full of nonsense. To determine the ideal sized toes, look at them in proportion to the rest of your feet. Reflexology encourages you to think 'out of the box' for a far more open and broad-minded approach to life.

Skin

When it comes to the condition of the skin on your toes, you are looking at the effect of your conditioned belief systems that influence your state of mind. Your skin changes constantly, giving you a fair idea of what is really going on beneath the surface. It *hardens* when experiencing difficulty in thinking in the same way as others; it *blisters* due to a conflict of interests; it *shines* when resisiting the opportunity to share bright ideas or when light needs to be thrown onto a particular situation; or *weeps* from being upset. Massaging the skin smoothes things over whilst, at the same time, gets to the root of what is really going on at a deep sub-conscious level so that any disturbing memories can be dealt with and eliminated for once and for all.

The colouring of the skin on your toes highlights the emotions that are linked to your innermost thoughts, showing whether you have loving, angry, hurtful, inconsiderate or caring notions in mind as seen in Chapter 08, p. 39. It's the essence of your thoughts that either enhances or drains your toes of their vibrancy. When more than one colour is seen on the toes at any one time, take note of the actual reflex that they are drawing attention to for further fascinating insight.

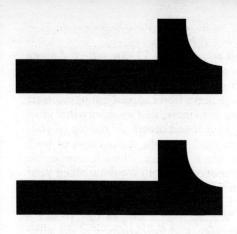

**your back
and neck**

In this chapter you will learn:
- about your arches
- what gets on your nerves
- how to relax.

Spine

The bony vertebrae of your spine (figure 11) are reflected along the hard 'knobbly' ridges of bone that extend from the inner joints of your big toes to just beneath your inner ankles. It's from your spine that all your nerve fibres spread out to infiltrate your whole body, filling you with incredible sensitivity that gives you the ability to feel for yourself and others. At the top of your spine is your midbrain, reflected onto the outer edges of both big toes, immediately above the bony joint, which is responsible for synchronizing all your movements and for controlling your breath and circulation since it contains both your cardiac and respiratory centres. Concentrate on these backnone reflexes for all *back* and *spinal disorders*, such as a *slipped disc* to put a piece of your life back into place, and for *curvature* of the spine to reduce the desperate need to reach out for additional back-up. Massaging these reflexes renews your sensitivity and reinforces your ongoing support and backing. Reflexology ensures the accuracy of all those messages being conveyed to and from your brain so that you can relax knowing that you are well supported.

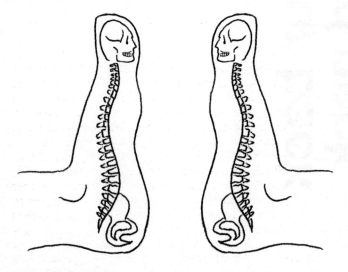

figure 11 divided spinal reflexes on both feet

The arches of your feet

The bony insteps that form your arches reveal whether you are 'in step' or 'out of step' with the general way of thinking and whether you have the inner strength to go against the 'norm'. Your arches are affected by everything that you 'put behind you' and anything that 'goes on behind your back'. This also where you harbour most of your memories, especially grudges or 'unfinished business', which is why they are affected by every step that you take. When you were a baby it's likely that you had flat feet since you were so completely reliant on others to do everything for you; that is until you had the confidence to 'stand on your own two feet'. Once developed the arches should remain stable and supportive for the rest of your life, but the reality is that this doesn't always happen. They fall *flat* and collapse when there is so much emotional strain that you can't take any more, showing how difficult it is to 'stand up for yourself'; alternatively they *over-extend* to provide additional support, particularly during exceptionally challenging periods, or when 'bending over backwards' to please others.

Reflexology is great at setting the record straight.

Nerves

Your state of mind reflects the content or discontent of your soul, which then affects the content or discontent of your body's composition. Nervous disorders are your body's way of telling you that your thoughts are 'getting on your nerves' and it uses specific symptoms to let you know what in particular makes you so uptight, since certain thoughts jog specific memories that can create absolute emotional havoc inside, which only upsets you even more. It's at times like this that you are likely to feel way out of control, really pressurized, extremely anxious or unable to cope which can then tip the balance one way or another forcing your body to either overcompensate, in an attempt to get on top of the situation, or to just give in, in complete desperation. Nervous issues stem from being irritatingly irritable, on the one hand, or not reacting at all on the other; or from being far too tolerant, at one extreme, or being completely intolerant, at the other. Sometimes they are a result of being overly sensitive or totally insensitive, or from your patience being tested to the limit. It's the extremes that can affect you adversely (see Appendix iv).

When you're under strain, your nervous impulses become distorted or traumatized, with the smallest irritation sending them off at a tangent, making you react badly. Sometimes this can be as bad as the memory that haunts you and interferes with your status quo until you do something about it and change your mind. In the meantime, symptoms of uneasiness or 'dis-ease' are likely to come to a head, since this is where bad things come from in the first place; namely a 'bad' thought. If you pay attention to what the symptom is saying, you can get an idea of the type of thought that initially triggered it off. For instance, *pain* is an outward display of a grieving, anguished thought; an *ache* comes from an intense longing to be noticed as an individual; *tension* stems from extreme anxiety, frustration, fear or worry; *nervousness* is the result of ongoing uncertainty that creates havoc in your mind; *infections*, *inflammations* or *high temperatures* come from festering dissatisfied thoughts; whilst *convulsions* erupt from fits of rage that distort the brain waves, throwing them way off course. Massaging your brain reflexes in the toes (p. 42) has an immediate effect on your nervous system; it instantaneously calms you down physically, mentally, emotionally and spiritually. The resultant inner peace eases your tension, relaxes your muscles and ensures that your brain cells, as well as your nerves, receive their full quota of essential life force energies so that you and they can function as they should for the overall benefit of your mind, body and soul.

Hands

Your hands are handy for handling life, manipulating situations and moulding ongoing events, whilst your fingers have a knack of dealing with the finer details. The reflexes for your hands are those soft mounds in front of your outer ankle bones, on top of both feet (figure 12), which feel like miniscule fists when palpating them. Their characteristics give away information on how well you believe you are coping: they *swell* when you feel overwhelmed at the enormity of all that needs attending to; they *sink* when you are fearful or dubious about dealing with awkward situations. *Blood vessels* also appear over these reflexes whenever there's extreme unhappiness about the way in which things are being controlled, or because of feeling so out of control. Massaging these reflexes helps you to get to grips with all that's going on.

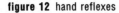

figure 12 hand reflexes

Feet

Your feet represent your stability and security, as well as your ability to step ahead and make progress through life. They are reflected onto the lower portions of both heel pads (figure 13), as well as onto the outer edges of both feet, just beneath the ankle bones (figure 14). Their reflexes *bulge* when life is perceived to be a drag or heavy going and they *sink* from the utter exhaustion of trying to get moving. When you massage these reflexes you are effectively giving a complete foot massage without even moving your fingers!

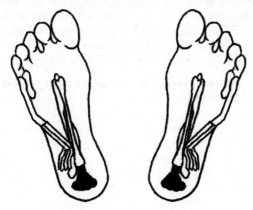

figure 13 feet reflexes on the heel pads

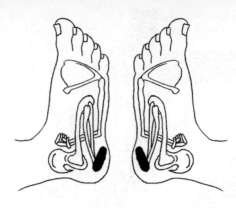

figure 14 feet reflexes on the outer edges

Complete inner calm

Massaging your toes and arches has far-reaching effects because of their relationship with your nervous system, which influences the well-being of every part of you. Reflexology effectively stimulates or soothes your nerves, which has an immediate impact on the corresponding parts of your body. More importantly, it encourages a change of mind and a much better attitude and approach to life. Remember that each set of toes has a specific role in ensuring your overall well-being: your *big toes* balance your intellect and intuition for the confident sharing of your innovative ideas; your *second toes* boost perceptions of yourself and others; your *third toes* inspire you to put your unique ideas into practice; your *fourth toes* help you to generate new concepts for a fresh approach to life, whereas your *little toes* expand your mind and free your thinking from inhibiting belief systems and social restraints, so that you can allow your extra-ordinary ideas to lead the way.

Life is an adventure of the mind that makes the impossible possible.

12

your big toes and toe necks

In this chapter you will learn:
- about your big toes
- about the influence of your hormones
- how sensitive you are.

Your 'thoughtful' big toes

Your big toes contain the main reflexes for your head, brain, face and cranium, reflecting those thoughts and ideas that are uppermost in your mind. They also reveal your intellectual and intuitive awareness, along with your spirituality and connection to your Higher Self. The usefulness of these notions for your well-being is picked by their related reflexes, namely your toe necks, thumbs, hands and feet to provide valuable insight into your nervous, endocrine, sensory and lymphatic systems, all of which depend on your approach to life for good health. The element that best suits your thoughts is ether because of its non-physical nature, whilst indigo, violet and blue, all with high, spiritual vibrations, provide an energetic link between your thoughts and the divine source. Massaging these toes offers you more space in which to be your creative self, whilst giving you access to the universal library of ancient knowledge and wisdom. Through reflexology your big toes can realign themselves so that they point you in the best direction to attain your soul's purpose on earth.

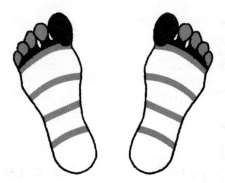

figure 15 your big toes and their related parts

In their natural state your big toes and toe necks act as superb spring boards for your thoughts and are the ideal means by which you can propel yourself and get ahead in life. The only thing that gets in your way is yourself! If you keep thinking that your own ideas aren't good enough, you hold yourself and your big toes back. This is generally because you feel far too terrified to stand up for yourself or because you fear the frightful penalties that come with being a non-conformist. Your anxiety, concern and worry keep tripping you up. The more you succumb to unsuitable belief systems and allow yourself to be conditioned into prescribed ways of thinking, the worse the situation becomes, because not being in control leads to a self-righteous approach and the need to be a control freak. Ironically, the more out of control you become, the more you try to control; a no win situation that can eventually drive you crazy! Nervous disorders evolve when things are 'out of order' in your mind and are definitely not to your liking; either because you are trying to be too much in control or because you feel completely out of control. Reflexology ensures that it's your unique ideas, and nobody else's, that propel you and get you ahead.

So take time to focus on what your big toes are telling you. They *bend inwards* whenever you side-step your ideas or try to put them to one side which can end up crushing your other toes as you succumb to totally unsuitable beliefs systems; or they *bow* in subservience when you keep trying to please others or are 'bowing out' of facing the world with your own extraordinary ideas; they *sink* into their socket when you allow yourself to be pressurized or are 'under another's thumb'; and they become *rigid* if you are too dogmatic or unforgiving in your approach because of having such set beliefs and ideas that are usually incredibly out-dated. Massage the big toes well for: *gout*, to reduce irritability; *itchiness*, *multiple sclerosis*, to be less strict on oneself and others; for *shingles*, to be less irate; as well as for all *nervous disorders*, especially those that literally stop you in your tracks. Reflexology helps to get your mind in order so that you remain well in line with your unique and special way of thinking.

Keeping your hormones in check

Although your pituitary gland is within the third zone of your toes, since it is situated in the centre of your head, being your master endocrine gland it relates more to all that goes on 'off the top of your head'. The best way to understand your endocrine system is to see it as the orchestra of your body, which joyfully maintains a harmonious inner environment and then sets the tone of your whole body. Your pituitary gland is well positioned to be the conductor, instructing all your other endocrine glands when to function, how to function, when to slow down, when to speed up and so on. Concentrate on these reflexes (figure 16): for *Alzheimer's disease* to elimate the need to escape life's harsh realities by leaving the mind. Also massage for *amnesia*, to erase the shocking memory from the mind; and for *bruising,* to calm inner turmoil and generate acceptance of all that's going on. Massaging these reflexes restores overall control and inner harmony for greater peace and general well-being.

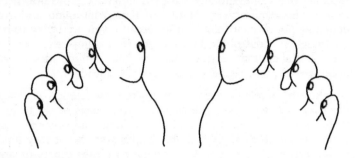

figure 16 pituitary gland reflexes

Sensory system

Your sensory system alerts you to what's going on inside and outside your body making you well aware of the interaction between the two. Those in the healing profession tend to be highly sensitive, which can be advantageous when it comes to intuitively picking up deeply embedded emotions and issues in their clients. Each of your senses affects specific parts of your body and is affected by a particular aspect of life, which is far more comprehensible when you know which sensory organ is related to which pair of toes and their related parts (figure 17).

For instance, your *inner sense* is linked, via your *thoughts,* to your *big toes* and *toe necks*; your *eyes* convey your *feelings* through your *second toes* and *the balls of your feet*; then *smell* and *sound* are associated, through your *actions* and *reactions,* to your *third toes* and *upper halves of your insteps*; *taste* is connected to your *fourth toes* and *lower halves of your insteps* through your *communications* and *relationships*; *touch* highlights how secure you feel within yourself, sensed by your *little toes* and your *heels*. When uneasy, you tend to become highly sensitive, which may distort the stimuli, either by magnifying them all out of proportion, causing a whole range of nasty reactions in your body or, alternatively, completely diminishing them into total insignificance, so much so, that, with no sensitivity, your body doesn't react at all.

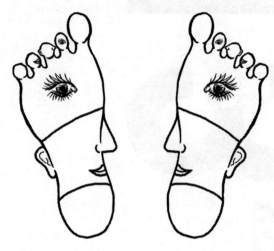

figure 17 sensory reflexes on the related parts

13

your expressive parts

In this chapter you will learn:
- how open you are
- about responsilibity
- about the need to be flexible.

Throat

The way in which you give voice to your ideas and share them with others affects your neck and throat, the condition of which is reflected onto the necks of each toe. The bony aspect of your neck represents your cervical vertebrae, which rebounds along the inner edges of both your big toe necks, whilst the actual back of your neck is mirrored across the tops of all the toe necks. Immediately below them, on their underneath surfaces, are your throat reflexes. Your toe necks reveal the impact of life force energies that enter and leave your body, as well as your ability to make your non-physical thoughts viable and acceptable in the physical world. Whenever you do anything with your ideas, their energy bounces back to you, which is how you learn more about yourself and the effect that you are having on the outside world. The condition of your toe necks depends entirely on the honest and open expression you have with yourself and others so that healthy relationships can be established. Massaging these reflexes not only makes you more open to the two-way exchange of life force energies but it also makes you more flexible by encouraging you to turn your head to see every point of view.

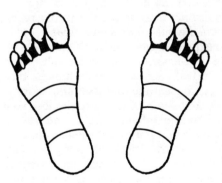

figure 18 neck and throat reflexes

Neck

When you allow your personal creativity to be strangled or stifled by social restraints, restrictions and expectations, it can lead to anger, guilt or stubbornness. The fear of voicing your own unique concepts and 'speaking up for yourself' grasps you by your throat and neck muscles, effectively choking and throttling you and your individuality. Your dread of speaking up generally arises from the apprehension of being ridiculed, along with the terror of the possible consequences, or even from a deep concern about outside opinion, or possibly from the trepidation of upsetting others. Any insecurity about expressing your own ideas and feelings tenses your neck muscles, thereby, reducing your agility, which can cause a pain in the neck. Meanwhile, if you believe that your thoughts are being threatened, your throat can go into spasm and you may even experience stabbing pains from continually 'getting it in the neck'. Extreme anxiety and uncertainty about talking out of turn but deciding to 'stick your neck out' can cause severe tension in this area. Concentrate on these reflexes for *cramps,* to ease the gripping fear of 'your style being cramped'. Reflexology makes you less twitchy by boosting your self-confidence and removing the fear of the dire consequences.

Neck and throat problems

When massaging the feet you may notice tiny *creases* and *wrinkles* in the toe neck area, which are indicative of strain, concern or worry about telling others how you really feel. Meanwhile *distinct lines* across the throat reflex are a sign of feeling *throttled*; whilst *lumps* and *bumps* could indicate either lumps of unexpressed emotion or alternatively swallowed tears, known as a post-nasal, which are a result of not being able to cry openly. In really extreme circumstances, this can cause the skin to weep. Concentrate on these reflexes for *sore throats,* to ease the pain and strain of trying to disclose your true feelings; for *laryngitis,* to calm inflamed, angry and frustrated words that are left unspoken and fester in the gullet; for *tonsillitis,* to open the way for the free flow of complete individuality; for *glandular disorders,* to enhance the distribution of lively thoughts and ideas for the well-being of the whole; for all *throat issues,* to dissipate the fear of any perceived adversity; also for *neck problems,* such as a *stiff neck,* to remove blinkers and open the mind. Observe the skin's colouring (p. 39) around your toe necks for further clues as to what is really preventing you from opening up and speaking your truth. With a concentration of lymphatic reflexes on either side of each toe pad and toe neck (figure 19), it's best to milk these well to remove any congestion that may be getting in the way of your free expression.

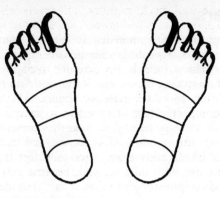

figure 19 facial lymphatic reflexes

Thyroid gland

Your butterfly shaped thyroid gland (figure 20) is reflected onto the lower, inner creases of both your big toe necks, mirroring a deep desire to spread your wings and fly, free of any constraints or restrictions. These expressive reflexes become *distended* when more time and space is needed to express your authentic self, whilst they *diminish* from the utter exhaustion of doing so much for others that there is no room for you. Meanwhile they may harden when there's little or no respect for your individual needs or when there's a resistance to your personal opinions. They may even develop an extra layer of skin as a means of protecting the little space that is available. Spend time massaging these reflexes especially for *goitres*, so that there is not such a need to reach out to others for their approval; also for *hyperthyroidism*, to create more space for the expression of the true self, and for *hypothyroidism* to boost confidence and re-energize the whole body.

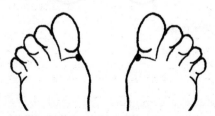

figure 20 thyroid gland reflexes

Shoulders

Reflected onto the strips immediately beneath your toe necks, are your shoulders, revealing your inborn ability to shoulder your responsibilities, which are actually negligible, since the Universe prefers to take the weight of the world on its expansive shoulders. Your shoulder reflexes (figure 21) reveal your willingness, even in the face of adversity, to carry on with your soul mission and overcome obstacles, as they present themselves on your journey through life. After all, they are 'broad enough' to carry your whole body from place to place! It's just when things become overwhelming for you, because you have taken on too many responsibilities, that your shoulders start to complain. They may *hunch* in defiance, refusing to take on any more, which may cause these reflexes to *swell*, or alternatively they may *give in* and *sink* under the strain or from the exhaustion of needlessly lugging around your hefty issues. Massaging these reflexes encourages you to let go of the overwhelming need to 'shoulder' so much, with the knowledge that the Universe is always there to give you a helping hand no matter what is going on. Your shoulders can then relax and move ahead with dynamism and fortitude.

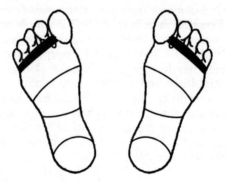

figure 21 shoulder reflexes

Wrists

Your wrist reflexes are immediately beneath the swellings of your hand reflexes under your outer ankle bones (figure 22), revealing your flexibility in handling the many differing angles of life, especially when it comes to dealing with others. Massage these tiny reflexes well for any *wrist problems*, such as *carpel tunnel syndrome* to ease any distress arising from the way in which life is being handled.

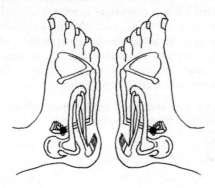

figure 22 wrist reflexes

Ankles

You ankles assist you in adapting to all those ups and downs that are invariably encountered as you progress through life. They rely enormously on your sincerity and truthfulness, especially within your relationships, to remain flexible and easygoing. Massage the minute reflexes (figure 23), on the outer edges of both feet, to enhance your ability to move freely, without any constraints.

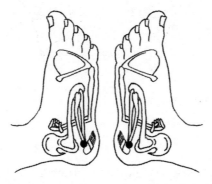

figure 23 ankle reflexes

So what do you think?

Reflexology reconnects you with your reason for being. It also creates greater awareness, so that you don't get so caught up and frustrated by the mundane aspects of life. In so doing, it encourages you to soar and reach unbelievable heights, particularly as your astonishing concepts take off. This allows your neck, throat and shoulders to relax, so much so, that you can really enjoy meaningful exchanges that create a much-needed balance and a deep inner calm.

Something you withhold makes you afraid and weak, until you find that it's yourself.

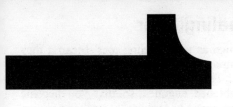

14

your second toes and the balls of your feet

In this chapter you will learn:
- about your ever-changing emotions
- how your feelings affect your eyes
- about your capacity to breathe.

Your second 'feeling' toes

Your second toes are known as your 'feeling toes' because they display thoughts of self-importance, your views on life and your opinions of other people. These toes help you to tap into the Universal source of enlightened energies, so that you become increasingly aware of a vast range of familiar, as well as peculiar, sensations, which you need to experience to know how you feel about yourself and others. Your spirit communicates with you through your emotions, reminding you of who and what you essentially are. Meanwhile your innermost feelings link you, through your breath, to all that's going on around you. This is how you create your own emotional environment.

Every time you inhale, you take in air, filled with the breath of those who are nearby, which can either be really pleasant and reassuring, or extremely stifling and disturbing. Once all these mixed feelings have been assimilated and processed by your lungs, you can then give a 'lungful' in return of whatever is 'on your chest'.

It's through your breathing that your second toes are directly linked to your respiratory system and indirectly connected to your heart and circulation. These toes are also energetically associated to your eyes, index fingers, the bottom halves of your lower arms and shins, as well as to your breasts and chest; the latter being displayed on the balls of your feet. Problems with your second toes highlight issues regarding self-esteem, invariably influenced by your father's circumstances, during your more formative years, and by your relationship with him. A poor *self-esteem* usually indicates that you feel that you never really met with his full approval. Squeezing the second toes can help you grow out of these distressing thoughts, with the knowledge that you can now make the changes that you wish to see.

Reflexology encourages you to come to like yourself and others better.

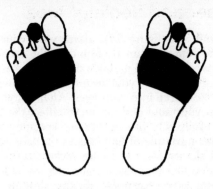

figure 24 the second toes and related parts

Emotions

The word 'emotion' comes from 'energy in motion', with the energy part being your thoughts and the motion part coming from their movement, as 'you run your thoughts' through your system. This arouses deep memories and unlocks suppressed feelings, which, once free, bring out the repressed, once-inhibited, aspects of your spirit which then gives you the impetus to act and react, according to what's going on, or not going on, in your life. Your e-motions are extremely powerful and, when used constructively, can inspire and motivate your spirit by evoking compassion, empathy and pure love. Emotions are such a vital part of being human and contribute greatly to your uniqueness and personal well-being.

The essence of those emotions that you keep well hidden is mirrored onto the balls of your feet. Meanwhile the colours that are linked to the way you feel are green and pink, whilst the element that gives your emotions free range is air. Everything that 'hangs in the air' affects both your internal and external environments. With any air in the body representing your emotions, be it through *belching* or *farting*, both of which are forms of emotional release. *Air embolisms* come from a gradual build-up of hurt emotions that eventually get in the way and bring things to a standstill. Reflexology allows you to relish the emotion whilst it is still relevant, but moves it on as soon as it is no longer of value.

> *Feeling good is your soul's way of shouting 'This is who I am.'*

Eyes

Your eye reflexes (figure 25), along with your pituitary and pineal gland reflexes, can be found in the second slivers that stretch across the central mounds of all your toe pads. They are ideally situated to make your feelings well known, especially to those who look deep into your eyes. After all, your eyes are the windows to your soul and, as such, reflect the true essence of your spirit. They help you to focus on specific aspects of life by adapting the multitude of light waves that come their way into meaningful shapes for you to see more clearly. Your eyes are energetically allied to your second toes and all its associates, making them very susceptible to any shift in your emotion. Every part of you is influenced by what you see or don't see, depending on how you feel at the time. Spend time massaging these reflexes for *blindness*, so that there is no need to 'turn a blind eye'; *cataracts*, to see the bigger picture more clearly; *coma,* to see the truth; *conjunctivitis*, to make things in sight more acceptable; *dry eyes*, to allow the flow of life; *glaucoma*, to ease set views, and for *tunnel vision*, to broaden the outlook. Rub the eye reflexes to open your eyes to the many exciting possibilities that are in sight.

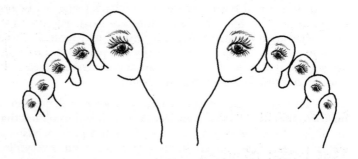

figure 25 eye reflexes

Your eyes reveal the antiquity of your soul.

Your insightful inner tutor

Although your pineal gland (figure 26) does share the same reflexes as your pituitary gland, it responds particularly well to the massage of your eye reflexes since these are the secondary access to them. Its production of melatonin depends on the amount of light entering through these optic organs. This is why the state and condition of these sensory parts are of utmost importance to your pineal gland's well-being. Through your eyes you pineal gland controls all your natural cycles, such as your mood cycle, sleep cycle and menstrual cycle, which are favourably or adversely affected by your emotions, as well as your perceptions of life that either make this gland work incredibly well or cause it to go out of control. Focus on these reflexes for *addictive* personalities, to get rid of the need to constantly escape because of not being able to conform and fit in, and also for *cancer*, to remove any growing resentment. Massaging the pineal gland reflexes eases congested emotions, making way for extraordinary insight and greater compassion for yourself and others. It also helps your mind focus, so that you can concentrate on what you are meant to be doing and become more intuitive and insightful with every cycle.

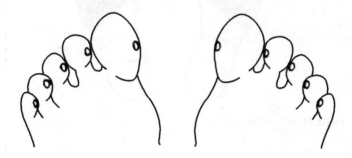

figure 26 pineal gland reflexes

The balls of your feet

The balls of your feet contain your chest, breast, ribcage, lungs, thymus gland, upper arm, airway and oesophagus reflexes, reflecting the impact that your feelings have on your personal well-being, which then determines how well you relate and respond to the constant changes and fluctuations within your emotional environment. The balls of your feet are naturally flexible, whilst their colour mirrors your ability to comfortably adapt and blend in to what's going on in your life. They put a real spring in your step when you feel buoyant, or they make life really heavy going when you aren't feeling so good. Give them a good massage whenever you need a quick boost to your morale. Also pay extra attention to them for *anorexia*, to bolster the flagging spirit; for *belching*, to calm inner panic; for *cancer*, to help resolve sadness; for *cysts*, to remove the need for pity because of ongoing misfortune; for *emotional congestion*, to relax the muscles for a free flow and distribution of life force energy; for *gangrene*, to restore the desire to be alive; for *pain*, to let go of feeling inadequate, and the hurt of being the subject of much criticism; for *snoring*, to finally be rid of deep seated emotions and for *wounds*, to heal injured emotions. Reflexology restores your belief in yourself and others, injecting you with such enthusiasm that you can't but help be happy to feel yourself again.

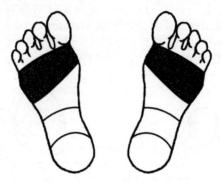

figure 27 balls of the feet

Your feelings vibrate throughout your whole being.

Fluctuating emotions

The constant variation of colours on the balls of your feet reveal fluctuating emotions. When memories flood back to the surface, it is those mottled pictures of past incidents that made you feel incredibly uneasy that show up the most. When massaging the feet, notice changes in colour as detailed in Chapter 08. The balls of your feet carry the marks of those heartfelt issues that have had the greatest impact on you, such as a *line* down the centre, when you are 'drawing the line' in order to survive, or are being torn by divided loyalties; *hard skin* and *calluses* may cover up all or part of this area as a form of protection when you feel particularly helpless or extremely vulnerable. Reflexology helps you to feel so much better about everything.

You can't choose how you feel, but you can choose what you do about it.

Lungs

Your lung reflexes (figure 28) occupy the bulk of the balls of your feet, both on top and bottom. They represent your ability to expand and become more of your incredible self as you take in big deep breaths to boost your confidence and, in so doing, know that you can confront anything that comes your way, regardless of the emotions that they could possibly evoke. You use your breath to suppress or express your emotions, whilst your lungs show your capacity to do this. If you keep interfering with the process, because you are not sure that you can cope, then the balls of your feet *enlarge*. If, on the other hand, you keep giving away too much of yourself, as a means of compensating for your perceived inadequacies, then they are likely to fall *flat*, leaving you winded and deflated. These reflexes often *wrinkle* with concern if you constantly worry about upsetting other people, even though you may be feeling emotionally distraught yourself. Excite the lung reflexes to give yourself the courage to become more of you.

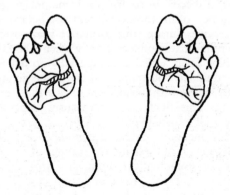

figure 28 lung reflexes

Breathing and respiratory problems

Breathing problems or respiratory disorders occur when interest in life has completely diminished or when you are feeling inadequate or unappreciated. They can also occur at times when you feel disillusioned or emotionally deflated. The temptation to keep heartfelt feelings to yourself, or to hide true sentiments behind a smoke screen, can eventually make it really difficult to take in air. Take time to soothe the respiratory reflexes, especially for *asphyxiating attacks*, to reduce the inner panic; for *asthma*, to remove anxiety so that it is easier to breathe; for *chest congestion*, to remove perceived emotional obstacles for the free flow of natural life force energies; for *emphysema*, for the encouragement to live life to the full; for *hyperventilation*, to create inner calmness; and for *pneumonia*, to allow emotional hurts to heal. Reflexology creates contentment within and, in so doing, ensures a more balanced and healthier relationship between you and those around you, which it does by filling you and your whole being with an exuberant appreciation of yourself and others.

Breast reflexes

Your breast reflexes (figure 29) overlap your lung reflexes on the balls of your feet revealing the amount of loving care you have to share which, in turn, determines the kind of love and attention you receive in return. Each mammary gland is filled with 'memories' of the mothering that you believe you received, or didn't receive, during your formative years. Remember, it is your perception that counts especially when it comes to this part of your body. Their actual size, especially on females, indicates how well equipped you think you are in the giving of yourself emotionally, along with the amount of care that you feel worthy of receiving. This fluctuates enormously, depending on how deflated or well boosted you feel. A *breast cyst* is usually a sign of deep emotional pain that has *accumulated*, by acknowledging and then letting go of these intense feelings of immense sadness, the growths of discontent can diminish. Caress these reflexes (p. 77) to nurture your body, mind and soul, as well as to make up for any lack of care, so that you feel good about yourself, regardless of what happened when you were a child.

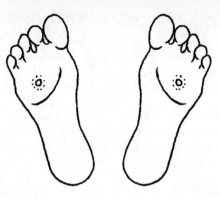

figure 29 breast reflexes

Thymus gland

The thymus gland reflexes (figure 30) are on the inner edges, halfway down the balls of your feet, where they represent the 'seat of your soul'. These reflexes may feel slightly swollen in the very young, the elderly and during times of extreme vulnerability, whereas they are more like hollows in every body else. Whenever you feel that others are constantly attacking you or being unreasonably critical, your thymus gland comes to your aid. Meanwhile any soul destroying circumstances can affect your thymus gland. *Swellings* over the reflexes are generally a sign of reaching out for more personal recognition; *hard skin* over them acts as a shield, especially when you feel defenceless or helpless from constantly attacking yourself for not being good enough. These reflexes tend to *give in* from the exhaustion of constantly having to be on the defensive because of ongoing emotional abuse and endless criticism. *Bunions* are indicative of trying to make space to just be yourself and are a futile attempt to break free from a stifling emotional environment that traps the soul and robs it of its individuality. Stimulating the thymus gland reflexes (p. 78) reconnects you with your true spirit. So pay extra attention to these reflexes for *aids*, to provide a relentless belief in one's uniqueness; for *bunions*, to free the soul of its many restraints; for *mastitis*, to alleviate the difficulty of so many emotional demands; and for any *thymus disorder*, to build up inner strength. Reflexology makes you feel so much better about being yourself.

Nothing is a threat, unless you allow it to be.

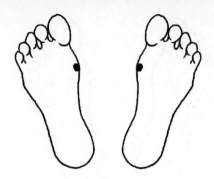

figure 30 thymus reflexes

Oesophagus

Your oesophagus reflexes (figure 31) extend from your mouth reflexes, along the inner edges of your big toe necks and the balls of your feet, to your insteps, revealing the courage of your convictions when it comes to following through with your decisions. Their characteristics are influenced by whatever is uppermost in your mind at the time, as well as your feelings about whatever it is that you take in on a daily basis. A ridge of *hard skin* appears over these reflexes when life becomes difficult or if you are trying to conceal upset feelings at being 'taken in'; they turn *white,* when you are tired of having things 'thrust down your throat'; *red* from the anger, frustration or embarrassment of having to swallow unpalatable situations and occasionally, they may turn *blue* from the hurt of being taken advantage of. *Flaky skin* indicates extreme irritability at becoming involved despite being unsure of what's going on. Coaxing these reflexes (p. 79) clears the way for you to move ahead with certainty, with the relief of knowing that you are back on track.

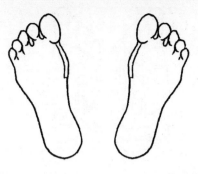

figure 31 oesophagus reflexes

Airways

Your airway reflexes (figure 32) extend from the bases of your big toes to approximately halfway down the inner edges of the balls of your feet, partially overlapping your oesophagus reflexes. Massaging these reflexes enhances the exchange of vital life force energies and opens you up to all kinds of incredible possibilities.

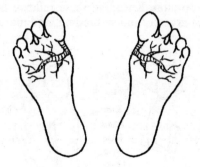

figure 32 airway reflexes

Elbows

Your elbow reflexes (figure 33) are those bones that are sometimes really noticeable because they stick out midway down the outer edges of both feet, revealing the amount of 'elbow room' you perceive that you need to be yourself.

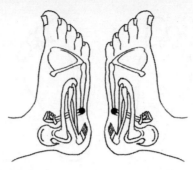

figure 33 elbow reflexes

Knees

The primary reflexes for your knees (figure 34) are situated in the centre of the balls of your feet, over your nipple reflexes, with their secondary reflexes (figure 35) being on the outer edges of your feet, between your shoulder and elbow reflexes. Your knees allow your body and mind to bend and change direction with ease so that greater progress can be made. Knee disorders often indicate that things are 'not in order' making it extremely difficult to give in or adapt to unwelcome changes or differences of opinion. Kneading these reflexes helps you turn the corner with greater 'under-standing' and more compassion.

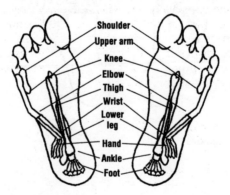

figure 34 primary knee reflexes

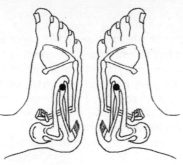

figure 35 secondary knee reflexes

Solar plexus

Your solar plexus reflexes (figure 36) extend from the inner edges of your insteps to the central hollows beneath the balls of your feet, although, in reflexology, they are mainly accessed through the middle indentations only. These are the most powerful reflexes on your feet because massaging them brings about an almost instantaneous calm throughout your whole being. Your solar plexus is known as your 'abdominal brain' and, as such, is favourably or adversely affected by your feelings about everything that is going on or not going on around you. This gives you a gut feel of what or who you should leave alone and what or who to get involved with. Too much or too little emotion really upsets it, causing its reflexes to either *sink* from emotional exhaustion or *swell* from being completely overwhelmed. They may also carry the *lines* of your inner turmoil or deep upset. Reflexology soothes any uncertainty so that you are far less sensitive and don't keep overreacting to distressing, nerve-racking situations, instead it creates an inner peace coming from the knowledge that everything is exactly as it should be.

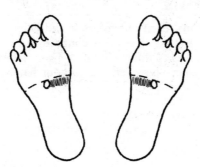

figure 36 solar plexus reflexes

Ribs

The reflexes for your ribcage (figure 37) cover a fair amount of the balls on your feet before extending around the sides and onto the tops of your feet. They reflect your capacity to emotionally reinforce and back your true feelings, based on what's going on on the sidelines, as well as behind your back, along with all those emotional issues that you have conveniently put behind you. They soon show whether you are 'getting it in the ribs' or when you believe that you have a 'thorn in your side'. The ligaments on the tops of your feet become taut from the strain of seeking extra emotional strength, particularly during exceptionally challenging times, or these areas may become puffy from all those unshed tears that you 'turned off' when you were told to pull yourself together. Massaging these reflexes gives you all the emotional strength and resourcefulness that you need.

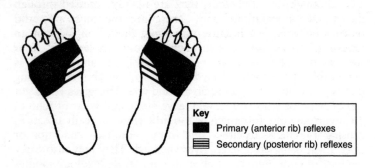

Key
■ Primary (anterior rib) reflexes
≡ Secondary (posterior rib) reflexes

figure 37 ribcage reflexes

Lower arms

Your lower arms reach out to assist and help you get through life, with their lower halves being connected to your feelings and their upper halves to your activities. These reflexes (figure 38) extend from your elbow reflexes to your hand reflexes on the outer edges of your feet.

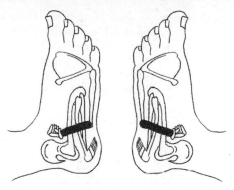

figure 38 lower arm reflexes

Shins

The lower halves of the shins are affected by your emotions, whilst their upper halves are influenced by your actions and reactions. Their reflexes (figure 39) extend from your knee reflexes to the feet reflexes on both outer edges of your feet, as well as on your soles.

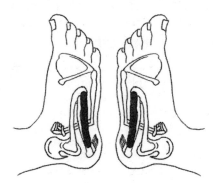

figure 39 shin reflexes

Upper thoracic vertebrae

Your upper thoracic vertebrae, which form your upper spine, are reflected (figure 40) along the bony ridges on the inner edges of the balls of your feet to reveal the amount of emotional support you believe you are receiving. When you are under a lot of pressure or, during really distressing times, these bony ridges may give in and appear *collapsed*, especially if there is little or no emotional encouragement, whereas they *bulge* unmercifully whenever trying to reach out for extra strength to get through particularly challenging periods. Soothing these reflexes eases the discomfort of feeling bewildered and encourages a non-critical acceptance of yourself.

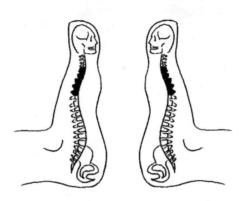

figure 40 upper back reflexes

Liberating the breath

Massaging the balls of your feet is a great way to set your spirit free. In so doing you are able to breathe more easily. Reflexology liberates the breath by easing tension in your rib cage, which allows your lungs to expand more fully, thereby enabling any trapped emotions to escape. You no longer need to feel so frustrated, bewildered or fearful, which takes such an enormous weight off your chest, with the resultant sense of relief being so overwhelming that you can't but help feel totally invigorated.

If you wish for kindness, you need to be kind to yourself,
If you yearn for the truth, you need to be true to yourself,
For what you give of yourself is always reflected back.

Your heart

Your heart is in between the feeling area and the active parts of your body, hence the saying, 'Do it with all your heart and soul!' Its reflexes (figure 41) are on the inside edges, where the balls of your feet and your insteps meet, with the larger reflex being on your left foot because of the angle in which your heart lies inside your body. As the centre of love and joy, your heart delights in nourishing and caring for all your body's cells but, in order to do this, it relies on the complete acceptance of yourself and others so that it can function at its very best. Distressing situations that 'tear at your heart' cause its reflexes to either *enlarge,* when you are constantly plagued by emotional issues or when you are reaching out for more love and affection, or alternatively *fade away* from having opened up and received precious little, if anything, in return. Miniscule *blood blisters* may develop over these reflexes when you are totally heart-broken or hard skin may form a protective shield against further hurt. Meanwhile a *cut,* when you are feeling emotionally cut off or cut up, may appear, for example, after a divorce or a separation. Caressing the heart reflexes encourages an incredible feeling of love and you are likely to end up really appreciating the gift of life.

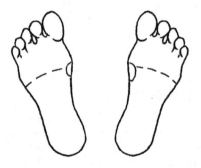

figure 41 heart reflexes

Blood and circulation

Your blood circulates from your heart to distribute love and joy to each and every cell throughout your whole body, all of which is so much easier when you are happy and relaxed. Constant unhappiness really upsets your heart and blood vessels, affecting their contents, increasing the possibility of heart and circulatory diseases especially when feeling a failure or when finding it really difficult to circulate because of a lack of self-esteem. Pay extra attention to the heart reflexes for *anaemia,* to replenish inner strength by boosting self-worth; for *arteriosclerosis*, to release the arteries from pressure; for *bleeding*, to replace deep sadness with greater understanding; for *high blood pressure*, to resolve unresolved emotional issues so that the blood vessels can expand and embrace new beginnings; for *low blood pressure*, to re-establish the flow of delight and enhance self-acceptance; for *blood clotting* and *cholesterol* issues, to open up the channels of communication so that they remain viable; for *heartburn*, to release the gripping fear of heart-rending issues; for *blood acidity*, to neutralize bitterness for good things to become more evident; for *increased white blood cells*, to naturally fortify the whole body when abused, be it mentally, emotionally or physically; for *leukaemia*, to release any unexpressed resentment at the heartlessness of it all; and for *varicose veins*, to strip out disagreeable and discouraging circumstances; as well as for all *blood disorders*, to ensure inner harmony and an unimpeded flow of joy. Reflexology re-establishes the flow of blood by giving you renewed passion for yourself and for life.

Circulation is life, stagnation is death.

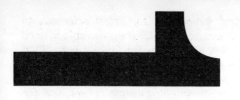

15

your third toes and the upper halves of your insteps

In this chapter you will learn:
- about the impact of your actions
- about the role of food in your life
- about things that influence your digestion.

Your third 'doing' toes

Your third toes (figure 42) are known as your 'doing toes' since they reveal all that you have in mind when it comes to doing something with your amazing ideas, the impact of which then shows up on the upper halves of your sole insteps. These toes are energetically connected to your third fingers, cheeks, ears, nose, top halves of your lower arms and shins, as well as your upper abdomen. They derive their energy, along with the rest of the body, from your liver, duodenum, pancreas, stomach, spleen and adrenal glands, all of which are affected one way or another by your actions and reactions, which, in turn, influence the workings of your upper digestive tract and its related parts.

The element that works in their favour is fire, which has both destructive and constructive qualities, symbolizing the need to get rid of the old before starting something new, whilst the colour they resonate well to is yellow, being the colour of intelligence and inspiration.

Concentrate on massaging your third toes and upper halves of the insteps for *influenza*, to flush out infuriating irritabilities; for *abscesses*, to drain away deep hurts; for *body odour*, to boost confidence; for *middle back problems*, to release any guilt that may have been 'tucked in the small of the back', with the knowledge that wisdom can be gained from all of life's experiences. Reflexology encourages your third toes to stand up for themselves and face the world with your brilliant ideas. Better still, it encourages you to run everything through your system so that something worthwhile is done with them; in this way, you can rediscover the substance that you really are made of.

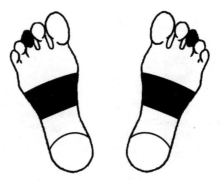

figure 42 third toes and their related parts

Nose

Your nose is reflected (figure 43) onto the middle segments of your toes. It works by taking in air to keep you alive, and also by detecting smells, which are the most evocative of all your senses, reminding you to 'follow your nose' and stay on track. Each whiff that comes your way is linked to a specific memory, be it a situation, person or event, which is why the mere thought of an aroma is enough to make you 'turn up your nose' in disgust, screw up your face up with displeasure or bring on a big smile of recognition. Then there are your nose characteristics, namely its size, shape and colour, all of which are linked to the acknowledgement of your achievements in life. Your ongoing successes depend on whether you can keep 'your nose out of other people's business', are being too 'nosy' or 'paying through your nose', which could put 'your nose put out of joint'. Reflexology heightens your sense of smell so that you can stay on track and achieve all that you came to do.

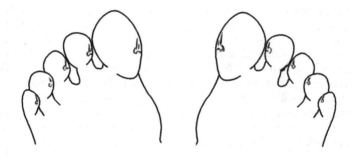

figure 43 nose reflexes

When things 'get up your nose' it's usually because you are a perfectionist and get highly irritated by the way in which others do things or don't do things, especially when they 'block your way'. Massaging the middle segments of the toes makes you more charitable and allows things to settle down long enough for the 'air to clear' so that you can change your approach. Concentrate on these segments for *adenoid disorders* to reduce irritability; for *colds*, to unleash a whole mass of exasperating circumstances that have 'got up the nose', clearing the way for new beginnings; as well as for any other *nose disorder*, for greater understanding and tolerance, so that you can concentrate on doing what you should to be doing. Rub your nose reflexes (p. 89) to help you truly recognize what an amazing individual you are, already having achieved so much in your life for the betterment of yourself and others.

Ears

Your ear reflexes (figure 44) are on the outer edges of the middle segments of your toes, representing your capacity to hear and really listen to what is going on or not going on. You have an inborn ability to transform sound waves so that you can receive direction, guidance and balance, especially from your inner voice. Problems arise if whatever is being said keeps 'going in one ear and out the other' or if it 'falls on deaf ears', which usually happens when constantly receiving an 'earful'. Working these reflexes helps you to open your ears, so pay extra attention to the ear reflexes for *deafness*, to replace fearful sounds and conversations of the past with greater discernment; for *earache*, to ease the pain of hurtful comments, which were either voiced or muttered 'under the breath'; or for *loss of balance*, to centre the mind so that both sides are given a fair hearing. Reflexology helps you to pick up and concentrate on important input so that you can move ahead with the sound knowledge of who and what you are.

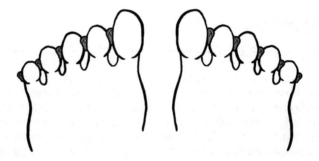

figure 44 ear reflexes

Cheeks

Your cheek reflexes (figure 45) bulge between the centre and the outer edges of the middle segments of your toes to reveal how coolly confident you are in doing something unusual that others might consider impudent. Rub these reflexes well, especially when feeling apathetic, to instil enthusiasm and re-establish a purpose in life. Give them extra attention for *meningitis*, to replace the anger and frustration of holding back with the determination to bring unique and unusual ideas out into the open, regardless of the consequences. Reflexology encourages you to do what you need to do, even when others try to stop you from being so different.

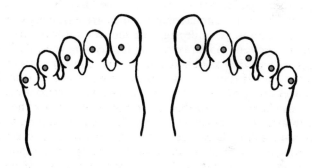

figure 45 cheek reflexes

Digestion

Your digestive process is immediately affected by a change of mind or a change of heart, as well as by fluctuating emotions that can range from extreme ecstasy to intense anger, from incredible fear to unconstrained excitement, or from severe nervousness to unbelievable confidence. Detrimental reactions from others as to what you are doing can cause great tension in this area, upsetting the harmonious expansion and contraction of your alimentary canal, which, in turn, hampers the progress of your food. This can cause much irritability and increased acidity, especially when you are feeling *bitter* or *resentful* towards yourself and others, which can then alter your chemical composition and also disturb your metabolism. Over time, extra layers of fat may form to act as shock absorbers, or as a way of preventing further damage from harmful attacks. Any of this can show up in the upper halves of your insteps, with *wrinkles* highlighting your concern, or *lines* revealing tight restraints, deep commitment or being tied up in something. Reflexology helps you to deal with adversity and encourages you to use it as an opportunity to get to know yourself better.

Liver

Your liver is reflected (Figure 46) onto the triangular mound that occupies the bulk of the outer half of your right sole instep, with a much smaller triangular reflex being present on the upper, inner quadrant of your left instep. Together they display your liver's lively characteristics, which are many, since it is the largest and most versatile organ in your body. It has a multitude of vital functions that are essential for keeping your mind, body and soul well energized and active at all times; even though the bulk of its activities take place whilst you are asleep. Whenever you feel frustrated or angry, especially about something that happened or didn't happen in the past, your liver 'takes the brunt' and its reflexes may become *distended*, particularly if you are hanging onto needless resentment; or they may *sink* from the utter exasperation of being so pressurized into meeting such ludicrous social and family expectations. Kneading these reflexes (p. 93) keeps your liver in a harmonious state, first by ridding you of toxic thoughts and noxious emotions, then by storing and rejuvenating your blood, so that you are constantly instilled you with passion. It takes your past to fuel your present, so that you can keep doing something really worthwhile with your life, whilst, at the same time, generating just enough heat to keep you comfortable.

Your liver is truly remarkable, just like you.

Your liver gets really agitated whenever you feel absolutely 'livid' because it contains most of your inner fury, profound dissatisfaction and suppressed guilt, which may erupt from time to time, making you aggressive, highly critical and foul tempered. Massaging these reflexes (p. 93) helps you to work through the past so that whatever happened is an asset, rather than a drawback. Spend more time on the liver reflexes for *burns*, to release the intense desire to retaliate; for *chills*, to stop you from withdrawing into yourself; for *colds*, to flush out old irritating notions so that exciting new concepts can come flooding

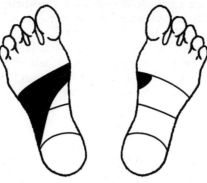

figure 46 liver reflexes

through; for *fatigue*, to fill your whole being with an enthusiasm for life that defies boredom and tiredness; also for *fever*, to encourage heated emotions to surface and then dissipate; for *infection* and *inflammation*, to 'put out the fire' raging within; for *boils*, to bring all those frustrations that simmer under the skin to come to a head, burst and be done with; and for *alcoholism*, to eliminate the need to drown one's sorrows by boosting self-acceptance; and for *hepatitis*, through greater understanding of what went on in the past; as well as for *jaundice*, to change jaundiced outlooks. Reflexology assists you in the realization that everything that has ever happened to you is exactly as it should be, since it's just what you needed, and you still need to go through, to discover the truth about yourself and others.

Gall bladder

The tiny rounded swelling of the gall bladder reflex (figure 47), based towards the centre of your right sole instep, highlights the joy or animosity of all that happened, or didn't happen in your past. If there's a lot of resentment then the bile is bitter, which could explain the higher incidence of gall bladder problems during wartime, especially amongst those who are forced to fight and kill against their will; the memory of these atrocities may linger for a long time and show up many years later as gall stones in their children. If there is accumulated unpleasantness, then the gall bladder reflex may possibly *harden*. Wheedle this reflex (p. 47) to coax any hostility out of you and to fill you instead with forgiveness for yourself and others.

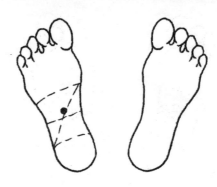

figure 47 gall bladder reflex

Forgiveness can't change the past but it can change the future.

Pancreas

Situated just above the 'waistline' of your feet, are your pancreatic reflexes (figure 48), which extend from the centres of your insteps to the inner edges, to reveal the amount of satisfaction and pleasure that you derive from all that you do, which is invariably based on the type of reaction and responses you receive from others. Problems generally start 18 months to two years after a really traumatic event that snatches away the opportunity to enjoy the fullness of life, usually because of not being able to get over what happened, be it a death, divorce, job loss, devastating move, serious accident and so on. The pancreatic reflexes *bulge* when reaching out for sympathy or greater fulfilment and can become quite *deflated* from the exhaustion of continually trying to please others to the detriment of oneself. Soothe these reflexes (p. 95), especially when life is just too overwhelming. Give them additional attention for *diabetes*, for past unhappiness to be put into perspective; *hypoglycaemia*, for renewed enthusiasm through greater appreciation and for *pancreatitis*, to ensure that everything is done with pleasure. Reflexology makes sure that your spirit is well replenished to the delight and complete satisfaction of your whole being.

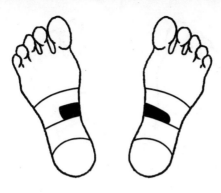

figure 48 pancreatic reflexes

Spleen

Your spleen ensures that you do everything with the appropriate amount of precision and attention to detail, so that you can attain the utmost from all that you do. Its small mounded reflex (figure 49) is only on your left upper outer quadrant. It tends to enlarge whenever there's an obsession or obsessive tendencies, especially when filled with outrage and revenge towards the family or society, whereas it tends to *sink* whenever tired of trying to abide by strict rules that seem so pointless. Palpate this reflex (p. 96) to bring out the very best in yourself and others, and also give it additional attention for *arthritis*, for greater give and take within the family and society; for a*ddictions*, to cure the compulsion to self-destruct by rebuilding a healthier self image; for *unhealthy appetites* so that a natural balance can be found when it comes to pleasing everybody; for *bulimia*, for fullness of life to be taken in without feeling overwhelmed or inadequate; for *obesity,* to help resolve weighty issues; and for *cellulite,* to stop self-criticism and promote greater belief in oneself. Also attend to these reflexes for *constipation,* to release burdensome beliefs that get in the way; *diarrhoea,* to bring to a halt the need to run away; and for *haemorrhoids,* to no longer feel encumbered, strained or suppressed. Reflexology gives you the faith to believe in all that you do so that, in the process, you gain greater appreciation of all those around you.

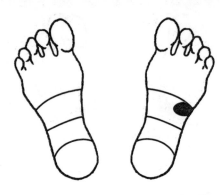

figure 49 the spleen reflex

Your behaviour follows your attitude.

Adrenal glands

Your adrenal gland reflexes (figure 50) are immediately below your solar plexus reflexes, with the right reflex being slightly lower and a little more central than the left reflex. It's these glands that give you the courage and resourcefulness to put your own unique and innovative ideas into practice, even though your way-out and unusual concepts may initially attract disapproval, adversity and criticism. These reflexes have a tendency to *swell* when overcome with fear, anxiety or terror or *sink* when feeling defeated and lacking the courage of your convictions, or when you feel discouraged from the pressure of continually having to prove yourself. Stimulate them well (p. 97) so that you have the audacity to do what has never been done before. Concentrate on these reflexes for *Addison's disease,* for a greater appreciation of personal assets, as well as for any other *adrenal disorder,* to boost inner strength and greater fortitude. Reflexology makes sure that you have the courage to do things differently, just because you are different!

Have the courage to live your life differently.

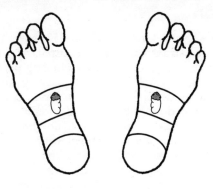

figure 50 adrenal gland reflexes

Cardiac sphincter

The reflexes of your cardiac sphincter (figure 51) are slight mounds that can be felt on the inner edges of both feet, at the junction of the balls of your feet and your insteps. As the muscular entrance to your stomach, it lets in food but stops it from coming back again, that is until overwhelming emotions get the better of you and literally make you sick, so much so that you end up nauseous or vomiting. When heartfelt feelings build up inside and make you puke, then *reflux* or *heartburn* are likely. Reflexology encourages you to 'stomach' all things that come your way, no matter how scary or difficult they may at first seem.

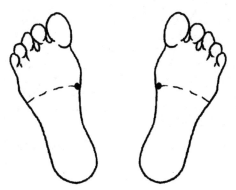

figure 51 cardiac sphincter reflexes

Stomach

Your bulbous stomach reflexes (figure 52) cover the bulk of the upper inner quadrant on your left instep, as well as a much smaller triangular area on the corresponding part of your right instep, showing how well you are 'stomaching' and dealing with your life. This is symbolized through food. In fact, everything and anything you do is linked to food; after all it is perceived to give you the energy to get on and do things. Furthermore, whatever happens or doesn't happen affects and is affected by food, be it your intake, your reaction, your likes or dislikes and so on. What really upsets your stomach is the unexpected, as well as any ongoing inactivity that creates deep dread, extreme concern or a fear of taking on anything new or unusual. Whenever you feel incapable of coping, it really disturbs your stomach, so palpate these reflexes well, especially for *abdominal cramps*, to be eased from the clutches of gripping fear; for *vomiting*, to make repulsive situations and circumstances more bearable; and for *peptic ulcers*, to stop gnawing feelings from eating away at you. Reflexology makes sure that sickness is seen as an opportunity to become stronger, since it gives you the guts to deal with anything new or unexpected. In this way, you can restore your belief in your personal capabilities.

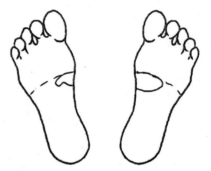

figure 52 stomach reflexes

When your body is sick and tired of all your moans and groans it will start to play up.

Pyloric sphincter

Your pyloric sphincter reflex (figure 53) is the slight swelling, beneath the balls of your feet, in line with the join between your second and big toes, on your right foot only. It's the muscular outlet of your stomach, which is greatly influenced by your ability to process all that you are having to deal with, based on what happened in the past. Fear causes it to contract, which can lead to *pyloric stenosis*, which is more common in male babies because it seems to be linked to the mother's unpalatable experiences with men, the thought of which still makes her sick. Soothing these reflexes provides you with the reassurance that it is okay to move on regardless of what happened previously.

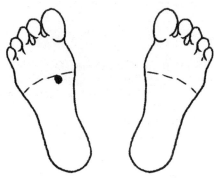

figure 53 pyloric sphincter reflex

You become successful the moment you start moving towards a worthwhile goal.

Duodenum

The C-shape of your duodenum reflex (figure 54) follows the perimeter of the upper inner quadrant of your right sole instep, revealing how well you are able to use the input of your past to make your present intake of life experiences work well for you. Your gall bladder and pancreas fill your duodenum with remnants of the past to assist you in processing every day events with greater wisdom and confidence. Massaging this reflex (p. 100) helps you to see how your past can be an asset in the present.

Experience is a hard teacher; it tests first and teaches later.

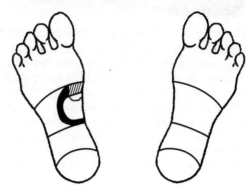

figure 54 duodenum reflex

Jejunum

Your jejunum reflex (figure 55) extends along, or just above, the waistline of your left foot, linking your duodenum reflex to your small intestine reflexes, depending on how confident you are about moving onto the next stage of the process. Soothing this reflex encourages you to keep going, rather than give up midway.

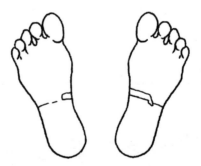

figure 55 jejunum reflex

You have to go inwards in order to keep going outwards.

Middle back

Your middle back reflexes (figure 56) are reflected onto the tops and inside of your feet, opposite the upper halves of your insteps, to reveal the backing and support that you give yourself in all that you do. It also mirrors any tasks that you have 'turned your back on' and shows whether you are 'bending over backwards' to please others. A *prominent bone* may pop up on top of your foot, from time to time, when you pressurize yourself to get things done; whilst *veins* frequently appear over this area, to show that the unhappiness of the past, or whatever is going on in the background, is being worked through to be got rid of once and for all.

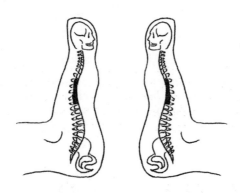

figure 56 middle back reflexes

If you do what you always did, you'll get what you always got.

Getting on with your life

There are many advantages to modern technology, especially since they take the drudgery out of mundane tasks that used to take up huge chunks of time, which frees you to get on with developing your creative talents. If, however, you ignore these opportunities and don't make the most of the time available, then you can literally make yourself sick. Your self-flagellating mind-talk really upsets your body because it knows that you are capable of so much more, so it draws your attention to the fact, through symptoms, that highlight your deep dissatisfaction, extreme frustration or intense bewilderment, in the hope that you do something about it.

However, it's not just about what you do or don't do; it's more about how you do what you do to make a world of difference for yourself and others. Life on earth is all about taking an active role in your life; living in the moment and focusing on what needs to be done in that moment, so much so that you remain empowered every step of the way. As you do so, you constantly expand your level of self-awareness, leaving you with little or no time to worry about what others are up to; after all they are entitled to do what they need to do in the way they need to do it, which, hopefully, is in the interest of all concerned. If not, then they must deal with the consequences. Reflexology helps you to be more considerate and aware of what you are doing, with the knowledge that whatever you do put out there has an uncanny knack of bouncing back and finding you!

Live well for today, for yesterday is but a dream and tomorrow a vision, but today well lived, makes every yesterday a dream of happiness and every tomorrow a vision of hope.

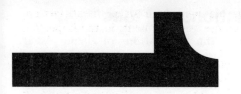

16
your fourth toes and lower portions of your insteps

In this chapter you will learn:
- the importance of relationships
- how to attain a balance
- why you need to be more discerning.

Your fourth 'relationship' toes

Your fourth toes have the reputation of being your 'communication and relationship toes' because they show how well you relate to yourself and others, which has a direct or indirect impact on your communications. The effect of this is mirrored onto the lower halves of your insteps, which, on their sole aspects, contain the bulk of your lower digestive tract reflexes, consisting of your small intestine, appendix and large colon, part of your excretory system reflexes (specifically your kidneys) plus some of your reproductive system reflexes (namely the fallopian tubes and ovaries). The energy of the latter, incidentally, is present in both genders. On their upper surfaces you'll find your lower middle back reflexes and also the secondary access to all the above parts.

Your fourth toes are energetically linked to your mouth, fourth fingers, bottom halves of your upper arms and thighs, as well as your lower abdomen. The element that connects them all is water, which ensures a good 'flow of conversation' and, if necessary, smoothes things over when you 'make waves'. Too much water causes *oedema*, should you be 'drowning' in the wake of overwhelming emotions whilst, conversely, your body 'dries up' and becomes dehydrated when you give too much of yourself to others. The colour that relates well to these parts is orange, a mixture of yellow and red, which brings out the vibrancy in everything and everybody, so that abundant joy and happiness can be gained from all your interactions, both internally and externally.

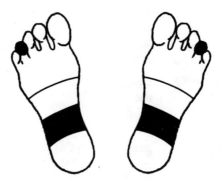

figure 57 fourth toes and related reflexes

Mouth

Whatever you say, be it in your mind or during the course of a conversation, has an immediate affect on you and all concerned; it is so powerful that it is enough to either make or break a relationship. The energy of your unspoken words occupies your mouth, affecting everything that passes through it whether it is entering or leaving your body. Any unexpressed energy immediately influences your food, as well as the air that you breathe, along with the words that leave your lips. Your mouth is an essential link between your inner and outer worlds, with the nature of all your interactions affecting your chemical make-up, either favourably or adversely.

On an energetic level, you intentionally attract into your life those individuals and circumstances that best mirror what's going inside you. This, in turn, influences the production of your digestive juices, with their efficiency depending upon the amount of give and take within your relationships. Every time you change your mind, the characteristics of your mouth change, either fractionally or quite obviously. Their reflexes *sink* when you are tired of the same old thing being said over and over again, or they can *swell* when you wish to 'speak your mind'. Your mouth, teeth, tongue and gum reflexes are all within the fourth portions (figure 58) of each toe, showing how well, or how badly, their influence reverberates throughout your whole body, the impact of which is picked up by the lower halves of your insteps.

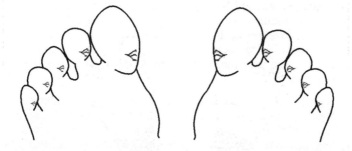

figure 58 mouth reflexes

When you open your mouth, try not to put your foot in it.

When massaging the mouth reflexes (p. 105) spend extra time on them for *halitosis*, to replace festering words with greater understanding, for *bleeding gums*, to restore confidence in decisions made; for *cerebral palsy*, for a more lively exchange of energy, no matter how bad things may appear to be; for *cold sores*, to bring some warmth into the situation; for *epilepsy*, to prevent 'throwing a fit' or 'biting the tongue' when misunderstood; for *gum disorders*, for the confidence to make your own mind up; for *neuralgia,* to ease the anguish of rejection or ridicule when being truthful; for *strokes* to bring to an end self-inflicted pressure to meet unrealistically high expectations; for *stuttering*, to boost confidence in sharing unbelievable ideas; for *tooth problems*, to take away the agony and pain of decisions being made or not being made; for *tinnitus,* to alert the mind to messages from the inner voice; and for any other *mouth disorders*. Massaging these reflexes helps you to speak your truth without the fear of what others have to say on the matter.

Begin by telling the truth and never stop.

Small intestine

Your small intestine is particularly interested in the give and take within your relationships. It knows what's good for you and should be 'taken on board' and what doesn't agree with you and so should be left well alone. Their reflexes (figure 59) occupy the bulk of the lower halves of your insteps to highlight the benefits that are constantly derived from your daily interactions, all of which are symbolized by food. Your small intestine helps you absorb the new for ongoing growth within your relationships since it is these refreshing energies that influence the development of your new cells.

These reflexes *swell* when you take on more than is manageable or *flatten* if you give too much of yourself, usually because of feeling fearful or lacking in self-worth; they become *dry* when feeling deprived or drained, and *wrinkle* with concern. Also look out for *crossed lines*, possibly from being at a 'crossroads' or at cross purposes or having a cross to bear, to mention but a few possible meanings; whilst *netted lines* may indicate feeling trapped, tied down or caught up in a relationship; meanwhile *deep vertical lines* could be a division or cut-off point, whereas *scattered lines* invariably indicate havoc. Then have a look at the colours (p. 39) to gauge your mood and emotional fluctuations.

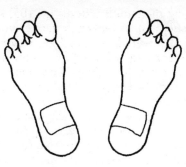

figure 59 small intestine reflexes

Massaging the small intestine reflexes helps to create a much needed balance in all your relationships, internally and externally. Concentrate on these reflexes for *bites*, to prevent biting remarks or from possibly being sucked dry; for *blisters*, to soothe any friction; for *candida*, to become more centered so that there's less frustration at being pulled in so many directions while trying to please others; for *fever blisters*, to increase tolerance so that heated emotions don't cause friction; for *cysts*, to relax the need to hang onto a mass of hurts; for *fungi*, to discourage old feelings from taking over; for *oedema*, to expel cumbersome feelings that are a weight on the mind, body and soul; for *parasites*, to evict those who draw on others; and for *malabsorption syndrome*, to replenish the whole being through an improved intake of data and ideas. Reflexology facilitates the absorption of the beneficial aspects of your life so that, by becoming wiser, you know how best to relate to others.

Whatever your role in relationships, the game is always the same.

Ileo-caecal valve

Your ileo-caecal valve reflex (figure 60) is situated in the outer corner of your right lower instep, representing the muscular connection between your small and large intestines. It facilitates the onward movement of anything that you no longer need to have inside you, otherwise it just ends up wasting your time and sapping you of your energy. Massage this reflex (p. 108) well because it is an exceptionally important one since it bridges the gap between what was and what is still to come.

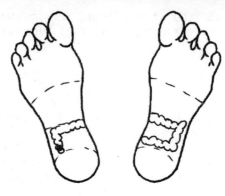

figure 60 ileo-caecal valve reflexes

When you discover how you function, you discover more of the world around you.

Appendix

Your finger-shaped appendix is considered by some to be surplus to your requirements. Its miniscule reflex (figure 61) is just below your ileo-caecal valve reflex on your right foot. The only time that your appendix really makes its presence known is if you are in a dead-end relationship or are furious that your life is going nowhere in particular. The infuriation of being in such an awkward position can make you so inflamed that should the situation get worse, your appendix may even burst. Massage its reflex well, especially for *appendicitis,* to replace the frustration

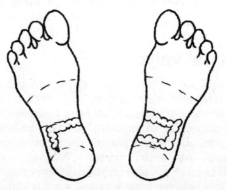

figure 61 appendix reflex

of being at the 'end of your tether' with greater empathy. Reflexology helps you to let go of anything that no longer serves you.

Bowels

The reflexes of your large intestine (figure 62), otherwise known as your colon, border most of your lower sole insteps and have four main sections: your ascending colon reflex, which stretches up the outer edge of your lower right sole instep; your transverse colon reflexes, which extend across both feet, just below their waistlines, rising slightly towards the end; your descending colon reflex that goes down the outer edge of your lower left sole instep; your sigmoid colon reflex which follows the boundary between your left instep and heel. The large intestine or colon itself contains the remnants of much of what previously happened in your life, which can bog you down if you allow them to loiter for too long. It mirrors your innate need to be recognized and acknowledged for all your accomplishments, which is why the transverse colon reflexes in particular can *swell*, especially when constantly competing against oneself and others because of never being satisfied, or when pressuring oneself into performing better than one's best, but often for all the wrong reasons. Cajole these reflexes to move on old thoughts and worked-through, worn-out emotions that would otherwise just waste your time and energy, otherwise they could possibly interfere with your current affairs and threaten your well-being. Give these reflexes extra attention for *colic* in babies, to pacify the mother's impatience; for *colitis*, to soothe

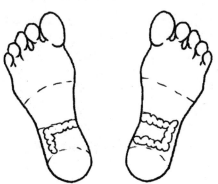

figure 62 large intestine/colon reflexes

the fury of being under constant pressure; for *colon disorders*, to help expel the dread of failure; and for *spastic colon,* to relieve the irritability of always having to be the best at everything no matter what. Reflexology encourages you to keep moving for ongoing bowel movements. It also reminds you that a little bit of pressure from time to time can go a long way in creating more of an urge.

Life is not given to be wasted and ignored, it is given as a blessing.

Female reproductive organs

Some female reproductive organs are reflected onto the soles, whilst the remainder are on the inner heels. They reveal how feminine attributes can be used to enhance personal relationships by adding the soft touch. Massaging these reflexes creates a greater acceptance and appreciation of the female role in the formation, accommodation and nurturing of new beginnings.

Ovaries

The ovaries reflexes (figure 63) are situated in the outer lower corner of both insteps, reflecting your ability to create and generate new concepts, not just in the form of babies, but also in shaping and developing ongoing ideas. These tiny reflexes feel like two miniscule water bubbles situated just beneath the surface. When menstruating, the reflex of the ovulating ovum enlarges, whilst that of the resting ovum virtually disappears. Since the contraceptive pill prevents ovulation it can make these minute reflexes barely discernable.

Swollen ovary reflexes usually indicate accumulated frustration, when you are bursting with novel notions but have no idea what to do with them, whilst *sunken* reflexes often indicate that your amazing notions are being ignored or that there is a possible conflict with another woman. Caress these reflexes (p. 111) to make sure that exciting new concepts are constantly generated to bring about much-needed changes to the world.

111
your fourth toes and lower
portions of your insteps

16

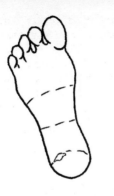
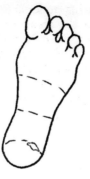

figure 63 ovaries reflexes

Fallopian tubes

The primary fallopian tubes and finger reflexes (figure 64) stretch across the soles, along or near the base of the fleshy instep, whilst their secondary reflexes (figure 65) extend over the ankle creases from one ankle bone to the other. They are responsible for making sure that the new concepts have a chance of being fertilized so that they can come to life. Soothing these reflexes makes this a viable and worthwhile proposition.

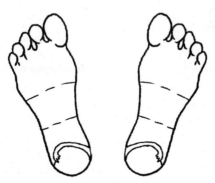

figure 64 primary fallopian tube and finger reflexes

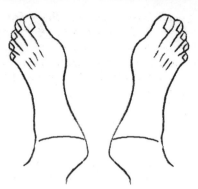

figure 65 secondary fallopian tube and finger reflexes

Kidneys

Also in your instep area are some excretory reflexes, namely these of your kidneys (figure 66) which are involved in the initial process of letting go of worked through thoughts and emotions that would otherwise overload you to such an extent that you would literally burst! These tiny kidney-shaped reflexes are vertical mounds, situated immediately beneath your adrenal gland reflexes, with the right reflex being slightly lower and a fraction further in than the left one.

They *swell* when you have to work though a mound of old thoughts and emotions; *harden* when you experience constant disappointments or feel really disillusioned and *sink* when you feel deflated or defeated. Milking these reflexes eases the process

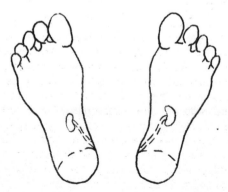

figure 66 kidney reflexes

of letting go. Spend more time on them for *nephritis*, to eliminate the anger and frustration of being constantly thwarted; and for *childhood ailments*, to discourage the parents from acting like kids. Reflexology helps you to flush away the past in the knowledge that life flows so much easier when there are no remnants getting in the way.

Ureter

Your ureter reflexes (figure 67) extend from the mid-point of your kidney reflexes to your bladder reflexes, revealing the internal flow of urine and your ability to move on.

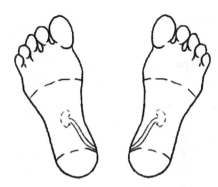

figure 67 ureter reflexes

Upper arms

Along the outer edges of the balls of your feet are your upper arm reflexes (diagram 68), which extend from the bases of your little toes to about halfway along both feet. The lower halves are affected by your communications and relationships, whilst the upper halves reveal your willingness to let go of those who need to be emotionally free of your clutches, as well as your ability to reach out and embrace new beginnings. These reflexes show how much space you believe you have to be yourself. They *swell* when you wish to break free from being tied to the family, or they develop *hard skin* to show how difficult it is to escape perceived obligations. Massaging these reflexes (p. 114) encourages you to release all those unnecessary emotional attachments so that everybody can enjoy their own space.

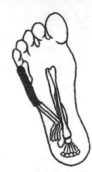
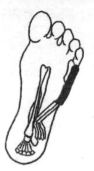

figure 68 upper arm reflexes

Lumber vertebrae

Your lumber vertebrae reflexes (figure 69) provide the backing for your relationships and also reveal all that is going on in the background. They extend along the bony arch from the waistline of your feet to just about the junction of your insteps and heels. These reflexes *bulge* when you are looking for extra back-up or *sink* when you don't think anybody is behind you. Massage these reflexes well to give yourself the courage to back yourself.

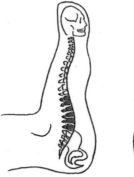
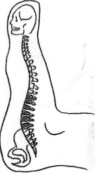

figure 69 lumbar reflexes

Digestive process

Reflexology calms down the whole digestive process making it so much easier for you to deal with daily events and cope with all that's on your plate. Circumstances become more palatable, your sense of taste improves, whilst challenging dilemmas become a pleasure to chew over, making them far more pleasurable to swallow and more gratifying to deal with. Your relationships become noticeably sweeter and you can really savour the delight of being with others. Massaging the digestive reflexes takes a huge weight off your mind and body and replaces it with a much healthier intake, a heartier appetite and a rush of renewed energy so that you can enjoy your life to the absolute fullest.

Think only the best, be only the best,
Do only the best, relate only the best,
Expect only the best.

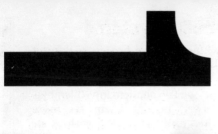
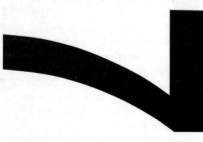

your little toes and heels

In this chapter you will learn:
- about the influence of family and society
- why and when to let go
- how to make better progress.

Family and social belief systems

The height and stature of your little toes show the impact that your family and social belief systems have had on your standing and status in society. When they are relaxed but upright and well-sized they show that you really do believe in yourself and are proud to be your own person, whereas if they *bow*, you tend to kowtow to your family and keep your true self hidden in the background.

Although they may be small, do not be misled by their appearance because they are energetically linked to your little fingers, jaw and pelvis, as well as your excretory, reproductive, skeletal and muscular systems. They have incredible muscle power when 'push comes to shove' which is why you need to get on in your own way, all of which is picked up and reflected in your heels. Your little toes and heels reveal how secure you feel about being yourself; the prouder you are of your achievements, the easier it is for you to move on and, as you do so, to grow and develop into the most unique and incredible individual that you are meant to be. Being so grounded, the element that they both feel most comfortable with is earth, which helps you to establish your roots, whilst leaving you free to come and go, as well as move on, should you so wish. The colour that inspires them is a deep passionate red, filled to the brim with all the energy that you could possibly need to get on with your life. Your little toes, along with your heels, balance your feet and act as shock absorbers, if necessary, because they actually prefer putting the 'spring back in your step', providing you will let them!

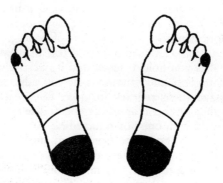

figure 70 little toes and heels

Heels

Whenever you limit yourself or hold yourself back it immediately shows up in your heels. They become *bruised* when past hurts get in the way; *crack up* when feeling divided or pulled in many directions; *harden* when experiencing difficulty in making progress; *heavy* when everything is heavy going; their rims become *tough* from constantly digging the heels in. Meanwhile *painful* heels indicate unpleasant growth experiences; *rough* heels imply that it's a challenge to make progress; *spongy* heels is a sign of giving in far too easily; whilst *insignificant* heels suggest a tendency to tread carefully and walking on egg shells. The colour of your heels reveals the emotion involved (p. 39). Rub your heels well to help you to expand beyond social restraints, so that you can move on without self-doubt, uncertainty or fear. Concentrate on the heels for *accidents*, to get rid of needless recklessness; for *calluses*, to bring out the 'true you'; for *fistulas*, to dispense with the need for additional emotional escape routes; for *plantar warts*, to let go of the frustration and change direction; for *rheumatism*, to release past resentment; for *ulcers*, for greater belief in oneself; and for *weakness*, to make it easier to move ahead and for all *muscular* and *skeletal disorders*, to provide the inner strength to enjoy the fullness of life.

Jaw

Your jaw reflexes (figure 71), situated along the lower edges of all toe pads, show how confident you are about the way in which you think. The solidity of your jaw provides a firm, yet mobile platform, for you to bounce off your own ideas, although its flexibility does depend on the amount of courage you have in 'speaking your mind'. Uncertainty and fear of what others may say often makes you hold yourself and it back, which creates a build up of tension and tautness that can adversely affect its joints. Massage these reflexes (p. 119) for greater flexibility. Spend extra time on them for *acne*, to neutralize inner fury at not facing the world with one's own incredible concepts; for *ageing,* to set the mind and body free from worn-out belief systems, so that the whole being can be revitalized and rejuvenated; and for *migraine headaches,* to release the mind from intense pressure; for *paralysis*, to deal with the terror of moving 'a-head;' for *Parkinson's disease*, to firm up the shaky foundation; and for all *jaw disorders*. Reflexology gives you the flexibility and confidence to 'open your mouth' and voice what's on your mind whenever there's an opportunity for self-improvement.

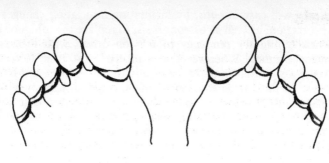

figure 71 jaw reflexes

Skin

The sensitivity of your skin reveals all that goes on 'beneath the surface' with its colour, especially on your feet, highlighting emotions that surface from time to time and change (p. 39) continuously, as your sub-conscious mind chatter hops from one theme to another. By encouraging a change of mind and a more tolerant approach to life, reflexology helps you to as well as alter the skin that you are in. When you are calm, you don't react so badly to everything that's going on around you, and you are less likely to let things get under your skin.

Skeleton

Your solid skeleton (figure 72) reveals the substance you are made of. It makes you aware of your resourcefulness, as well as all that it has in store for you on your journey through life. Your skeletal reflexes are extensively mapped out throughout both feet and provide vital clues as to how secure you are about being yourself. The *stronger* your bones, the greater your confidence, which makes you feel really good about yourself, whereas *weak* bones can barely hold you upright because you don't believe enough in yourself and therefore lack the strength and resourcefulness to keep going, which is usually at times that you believe your stuffing has been knocked out of you. *Breaking a bone* can often confirm the need to break away, with the position providing the clue as to what or who to break away from. Massaging your feet helps you to break away from limiting circumstances and it also prevents *bone deformity,* by liberating your mind from the perceived pressures of having to bow and bend into unsuitable belief structures. Massaging these reflexes will ease *bursitis*, by facilitating infuriating changes in the direction; as well as *osteoporosis*, to replace the 'oh poor us' mentality and the tendency to rely on others with increased inner substance. Wherever bones protrude on your feet it is usually a sign that more space or additional support and back-up are needed; again note where it is to get an idea of what's going on. Reflexology is an excellent way to bolster your inner strength and replenish your resourcefulness. It helps you to make the most of adversity, by using it as a guideline to sketch out another plan, especially when the present one isn't going anywhere in particular.

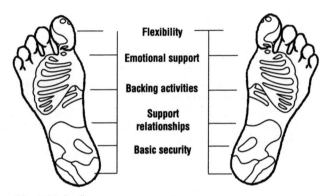

figure 72 skeletal reflexes

Muscles

It's thanks to the flexibility and adaptability of your muscles (figure 73) that you are able to expand every time you implement your innovative concepts, which, in turn, helps you to grow and develop into the person you are meant to be. The more open-minded you are, the more flexible your muscles are! Meanwhile very set beliefs and fear make them taut, rigid and, sometimes, unforgiving. Reflexology encourages you to extend beyond self-imposed limitations, giving your muscles the opportunity to stretch themselves with ease so that you have the capacity to put your way-out and extraordinary thoughts into action. They also give your feet the strength, tone, power and impetus so that you can take the next step towards self-empowerment. Your muscles love to be soothed and respond exceptionally well to being massaged.

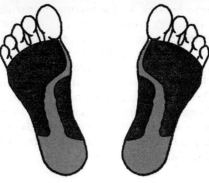

figure 73 muscular reflexes

Pelvic bone

Your pelvic bone reflexes (figure 74) occupy most of your heel pads and their surrounding areas. Their solid foundation allows you to pivot, especially when changing direction, and to energetically stride out for greater personal progress, as well as ongoing advancement.

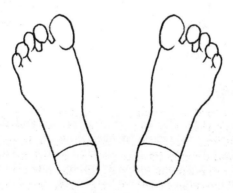

figure 74 pelvic bone reflexes

The joy of your spirit indicates its strength.

Hips

Your body is propelled through life by your hips, which give you the motivation and incentive to move ahead and get going. These prominent bones are reflected onto both outer ankle bones (figure 75), whilst the small firm swellings, just beneath them, reflect the ball and socket joints at the tops of your legs. Together they reveal your ability to move forwards, backwards or sideways. They *swell* when feeling overburdened or weighed down and develop *broken blood vessels* when unhappy at the lack of progress. Massaging these reflexes helps you change direction with greater ease and understanding.

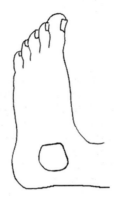

figure 75 hip reflexes

Buttocks

Your buttocks are the seat of your power and their reflexes (figure 76) on your rounded heels beneath your outer ankle bones, reflect the amount of command that you have over your direction in life. *Flabby buttocks* imply a lack of control from being so reliant on others for basic security, whilst exceptionally *taut buttocks* suggest someone who keeps an extremely tight rein and firm control over all their affairs, especially the purse strings. Massaging the buttock reflexes (p. 123) helps you to empower your true self so that it can come to the forefront and be noticed.

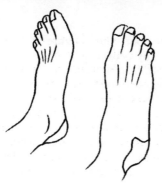

figure 76 buttock reflexes

Rectum

Your arc-shaped rectum reflexes (figure 77) are on the inner surfaces of both heels and represent your ability to finally let go of anything that's a waste of time and energy. It also reveals your willingness to release the rougher aspects of life, so that you no longer need to entertain them in your mind or your body. These reflexes may *swell* when *constipated*, when 'fear-full' of letting go; or they sometimes *sink*, due to being on the run, to escape current circumstance usually through *diarrhoea*; they may turn *red*, possibly from *haemorrhoids* and a fear of deadlines; or *distend* with *red* tinges, when there's a likelihood of *diverticulitis*. Milking these reflexes helps to alleviate any discontent at being unnecessary encumbered, strained or suppressed; whilst reflexology provides you with ongoing relief from carrying a load of 'non-sense'.

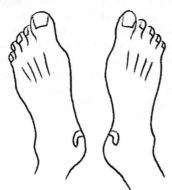

figure 77 rectum reflexes

Anus

The reflexes for your anus (figure 78) are small palpable indentations, midway between your inner ankles bones and tips of your inside heels. Soothing these reflexes rids you of the need to be so crude when you feel really frustrated from hanging on to something for far too long.

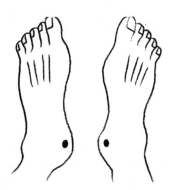

figure 78 anus reflexes

Bladder

Your bladder reflexes (figure 79) are the fleshy mounds on the inside edges of your insteps, at their junction with your heels. They reflect your bladder's ability to act as a reservoir for your worked through thoughts and emotions, until such time that you are ready to let go. These reflexes can *swell* quite considerably especially when you are unhappy with your intimate partner. Gently caress these reflexes (p. 125) so that you are more accommodating of your partner's downfalls. Give the bladder reflexes extra care for *cystitis* and any other *bladder disorder*, to expel old concerns that play havoc with your emotions. Reflexology helps your bladder to feel more relaxed so that it can release every last drop when it comes to it.

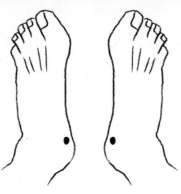

figure 79 bladder reflexes

Urethra

Your urethra reflexes extend from the fleshy mounds on the inner aspects of your feet to the slight indentations, midway between the inner ankle bones and tips of the heels, if you are female (figure 80), and to the very tips of the heels, should you be male (figure 81). Your urethra consists of two muscular sphincters that control the final release of all your old worked through energies. This ability is temporarily lost when you are fearful, under extreme pressure or in a particularly life-threatening situation that could usurp your position and status in life, over which you believe that you have no control. This can lead to *incontinence* in the elderly or *bed wetting* in youngsters, the latter being due to tension at home because of the father's circumstances. Massaging these reflexes helps you to regain control of the comings and goings within your mind so that you can physically go with the flow.

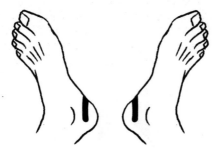

figure 80 female urethra reflexes

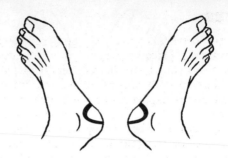

figure 81 male urethra reflexes

Lower reproductive parts

The reflexes for your lower reproductive organs and glands (figure 82) are reflected onto the inner triangular areas of your heels, representing your masculine and feminine traits, of which you have both. Your male energy comes from your father's sperm and your female energy from your mother's egg, which is why your reproductive organs represent all that goes with being either a male or a female. These reflexes look *bruised* when either hurt from being taken advantage of, or from not receiving recognition because of being a specific gender, whilst they develop small broken blood vessels when intensely unhappy at perceived mental, emotional, physical or spiritual gender abuse. Reflexology brings about the realization that there are no 'opposites', only 'oppo-sames', with each gender being reliant on the presence of the other for the balance in life. One without the other would bring life to a standstill.

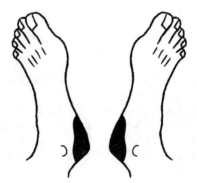

figure 82 reproductive reflexes

Uterus

The uterus, better known as the womb, reflects your home; after all it was the place in which you first resided from your conception to your birth. Its reflexes (figure 83), on the lower inside edges of both insteps, reflect the female principle and reveal all that is happening or not happening within the home environment. They *swell* during pregnancy with new concepts, or a baby; turn *red* when disappointed or frustrated at the lack of acceptance or recognition of creative notions; look *battered* when unable to get ahead because of social beliefs; or develop a *cut,* indicating a severance of home ties or it could indicate a *hysterectomy.* Concentrate on massaging these reflexes for any *menstrual disorder,* to create a more favourable environment in which women are appreciated and can enjoy all that being a female entails. Reflexology helps to make the home environment more relaxed, so that everybody feels well loved and adequately nurtured.

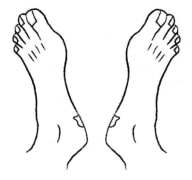

figure 83 uterus reflexes

Vagina

The vagina reflexes (figure 84), on the hollows between the inner ankle bones and heel tips, reveal the reaction at having to meet social obligations, along with all that comes with being a female. *Broken blood vessels* or *bruising* over these reflexes can be indicative of sexual abuse, be it physical, mental or emotional. Massaging these reflexes (p. 128) creates an inner pride at being a women.

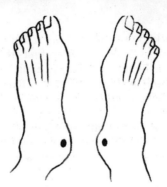

figure 84 vagina reflexes

Male reproductive organs

The male reproductive organs and glands are situated on the inside heels of both feet (figure 85), reflecting a man's perception of himself and his feelings regarding his designated role in life. They reveal how well he functions when needing to rise to the occasion and perform his manly duties. Spend extra time on these reflexes for male issues, such as *impotence*. Reflexology helps men to realize that they don't have to be a 'men-ace' to get their point across and that it is okay to just be their charming selves!

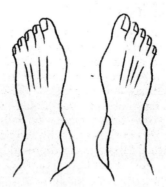

figure 85 male reproductive reflexes

Testes

The position of the testes reflexes (figure 86) is not always the same because they have the tendency to hang lower down when it's hot, to help them cool down, whilst making a hasty retreat back to the body, in search of some warmth, as soon as it gets too cold. The testes continually 'test their way' through life. Their sperm count is symbolic of their perceived ability to make a worthwhile contribution to society's progress. Stimulating the reflexes helps them get on and do what they need to do, and be proud of being a man.

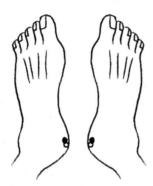

figure 86 testes reflexes

The base of your back

The solid reflexes of your lower back (figure 87) are the sections of your bony insteps that curve underneath your inner ankle bones. They reflect the amount of basic backing and support that you believe you have when it comes to expanding your horizons and exploring new territories. These reflexes *distend* when more backing, especially financial, is sought, and they *sink* when there's insufficient money or a drain on personal resources. Bolster these reflexes (p. 130) to reinforce your belief in your own worth. Massage them thoroughly for *lower back pain*, to relieve the hurt at not having the back up needed to get on. Reflexology enriches your mind, body and soul to such an extent that you soon realize you have everything you need at your disposal, especially when you ask the universe for assistance and support.

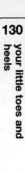

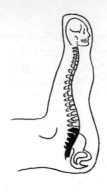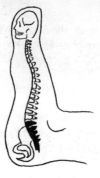

figure 87 lower back reflexes

*Life can be understood backwards, but must be lived
forwards!*

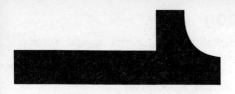

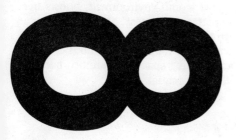

18

pregnancy

In this chapter you will learn:
- about reflexology's role in pregnancy
- about the benefits to all concerned
- how to detect a baby's presence.

Before conception

Before falling pregnant, ideally both parents should receive reflexology on a regular basis, for at least a year beforehand. For the father-to-be it helps ensure stronger, healthier sperm and prepares him physically, mentally, emotionally and spiritually, so that he has the inner strength and confidence to support the mother-to-be throughout the pregnancy. For the mother-to-be it creates a much more conducive womb environment, boosts her resourcefulness, gives her greater awareness of her role as a mother and increases her intuitive abilities, all of which makes the unborn baby feel most welcome. With her womb being so receptive and providing such a loving space, the unborn baby is able grow and develop to its full potential.

During pregnancy

During pregnancy the reproductive reflexes enlarge or form a shadow in the shape of the developing embryo (figure 88) around six weeks after conception. This embryonic shape can often be seen in the uterine reflex on the inside of one or both feet. In 80 per cent of pregnancies, if the swelling is on the right instep, the baby is usually a boy, and, if it's on the left foot, it is more likely to be a girl, although this is by no means a totally accurate prediction.

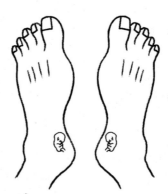

figure 88 around six weeks of pregnancy

Both the mother-to-be and her unborn baby thrive on reflexology, whilst the father-to-be gains greater understanding of what's going on so that he knows what to do and when to do it. For pregnant women, your touch should be exceptionally gentle, light and loving, particularly over her womb reflexes. Spend time caressing her breast, uterus, pelvis and vagina reflexes to allow them all to undergo natural changes with ease. Ideally, if the father-to-be gives his partner reflexology, he is likely to feel more involved and is able to contribute something really worthwhile to the process. It also establishes a much healthier relationship between the two, as well as a bond with the unborn baby. Massaging the mother-to-be's feet helps to deal with *morning sickness,* by reassuring her that she can and will cope; it eases any *back pain* by giving her greater inner strength; it prevents or soothes *varicose veins* by ensuring that her journey is pleasurable; and it enhances the *blood flow,* especially to her womb, so that there is a good supply of vital life force energies being received by the developing baby. Most importantly, it keeps her well, content and happy.

As the developing baby becomes more noticeable in the body, its outline is likely to become increasing evident on the corresponding parts of the feet, which, at times, can be so clear that it's possible to determine the various body parts, particularly its head and buttocks (figure 89). If the baby is in a breech or unnatural position, try rotating the mother-to-be's little toes, since this can encourage the unborn baby to turn. Reflexology makes sure that both the mother-to-be and unborn baby are well cared for, so that they feel completely at home with one another.

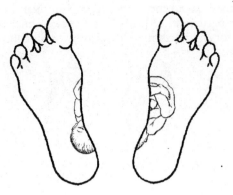

figure 89 reflection of the developing foetus

During childbirth

As soon as the baby's head engages in the pelvic cavity, small rounded swellings can often be seen on the edges of the heels of both feet, near the insteps (figure 90).

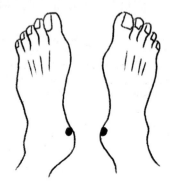

figure 90 engaged head of the developing foetus

Giving reflexology during childbirth is excellent, especially when it's the father-to-be doing it! It calms, relaxes and reassures the mother-to-be, whilst engaging the expectant father, keeping him well occupied so that he feels that he can be of some use, instead of just standing around helplessly. With the mother-to-be being so much more relaxed, she is able to breathe more easily and more deeply, as well as give birth more effortlessly. Sometimes, even when her cervix is fully dilated, she may not be ready to push; the sign to look for is when her big toes draw back and all her other toes extend forwards (figure 91), then she is prepared to actively participate. All in all, reflexology makes the whole experience of childbirth more enjoyable for all concerned.

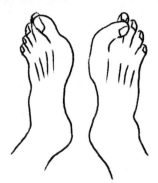

figure 91 mother-to-be ready for active participation in the childbirth process

After childbirth

When both parents continue to receive reflexology after their baby has been born, they remain far more relaxed and stay much calmer, which is exceptionally reassuring for the baby. The baby then has less reason to cry, with no distressing signals coming from either parent.

Babies love having their feet massaged, especially whilst being fed, and their tiny feet are well positioned when they are safely cradled in their mother's arms. Reflexology helps the whole family to adapt to their exciting new circumstances, which ensures a loving, homely environment, filled with complete appreciation for one another.

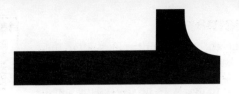

9

the technique

In this chapter you will learn:
- four simple movements
- the pressure to use
- the effects of each.

Four simple movements

There are four simple movements, which can be adjusted to meet the ever-changing needs of the recipient, so that every treatment can be personalized to suit his or her individual needs. The four techniques are the *rotation* technique, which forms an energetic link with the universe; the *caterpillar* movement, which improves the physique through greater inner strength; the *stroking* or *milking* method that soothes emotions so that the individual can feel better about themselves and others; and the *feather* or *healing* caress which reacquaints the recipient with their true spirit. Knowing exactly how much pressure to apply is an intuitive process that cannot be taught. You will just know when to be firm, or when to pull back until you virtually have no physical contact. To get a feel for these movements, try practising them on your hand first so that you can gain the confidence to do it on others.

Technique 1 – rotation

Gently rest the tip of any digit onto the reflex (figure 92) and apply slight pressure; hold for a while, and then very slowly release. A delightful tingling sensation may be felt as energy floods back into this area. Without moving your digit, gently gyrate it on the point of contact and keep doing this for as long as necessary. Now allow your digit to rest very lightly on the skin's surface for a short while before moving it onto the next reflex. This rotation technique is ideal for opening up and activating all energy channels, soothing fraught nerves and creating greater awareness of oneself and others whilst, at the same time, balancing and harmonizing the whole being.

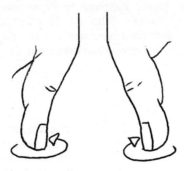

figure 92 rotation technique

Technique 2 – caterpillar

Place the *tip* of your thumb gently onto the reflex and then slowly lower your thumb onto its *pad* (figure 93) 'jerking it' fractionally forward. Now raise your thumb up onto its *tip* again before 'dropping' it back down onto its pad. Keep rocking your thumb, up and down, as you gradually move it, bit by bit, either *backwards*, to unravel the past, or *forwards,* to ensure that progress is made. 'Walking' the thumbs, in this way, eases muscular tension, relieves physical distress and alleviates aches and pains, whilst, at the same time, encouraging an improved approach to life.

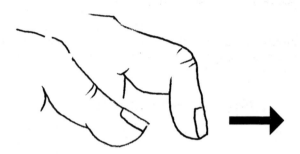

figure 93 caterpillar movement

Technique 3 – stroking or milking

Stroke or milk the reflex, after the rotation and caterpillar movements, by placing both your thumbs on the skin's surface. Now make long, reassuring and soothing sweeps (figure 94) over the reflexes, whilst applying slight pressure, as though gently squeezing a tube of toothpaste. This stroking or milking method soothes disturbed emotions, eliminates disruptive feelings, boosts self-confidence and creates inner harmony.

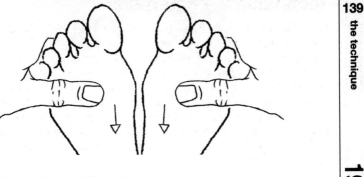

figure 94 stroking or milking method 1

Alternatively do this technique by moving thumb over thumb in shorter caressing movements (figure 95).

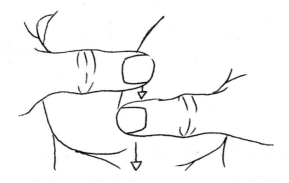

figure 95 stroking or milking method 2

Technique 4 – feathering or healing caress

This is the final movement of each sequence. Very lightly stroke the skin's surface, as though you are caressing the energies just above the skin's surface, by alternating your digits (figure 96), either in generous scoops or miniscule caresses. These movements reconnect the spirit with its soul purpose and bring the recipient's true essence to the fore, helping them to get to know themselves and others better.

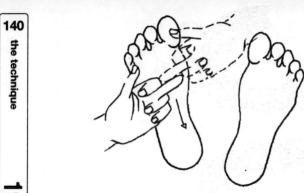

figure 96 feathering or healing caress

Your soul came to earth for the richest experience, not the poorest, for the most, not the least.

20

what to expect

In this chapter you will learn:
- about the sensations you will feel
- about less common reactions
- about pleasurable after-effects.

The sensations experienced

As the recipient drifts into the exquisite alpha level of consciousness, they remain acutely aware of everything that is going on around them, but they are so pleasantly detached that they really couldn't care less! In this way, they never need to lose control, despite appearing to be in a deep sleep. With their mind and body being so still, they can fully appreciate the fantastic sensations felt during the reflexology massage. Everybody's experience is totally different, which is why it is impossible to predict how your recipient is going to react. Being aware of what could happen, helps put their mind at rest, so that they can confidently let go and benefit more fully from all that reflexology has to offer.

Some of the more common responses are *heat loss,* as the body relaxes and let's off steam; extreme *tenderness,* despite the tender touch, as hurt feelings surface; a *sinking feeling,* as their mind and body drop off into a space of peace; a *floating sensation,* as burdens dissipate and a weight is taken off their whole being; *twitching* and *jerking* as a sudden surge of energy reaches previously deprived, tense areas; *pins and needles* or *numbness* in the hands when letting go of the dread of handling certain circumstances; *snoring* as deeply suppressed emotions finally escape; visions of *colours,* ranging from subdued, subtle hues to gorgeous bright tints, even though the eyes are closed.

Less common reactions

Less common reactions include *plucking* hand movements, when uncertain about how to handle current circumstances; *out-of-body* experiences, as the soul temporarily leaves the body for a different view point; *recall* of previous life situations; *singing* out loud. Some may even get the feeling that a murky lining of *emotional trash* is being pulled from their insides, like a piece of material. Just remember that whatever happens, it is absolutely ideal for the individual concerned; no matter how peculiar or unexpected it may be.

Whilst the feet are being massaged, the breathing can become so shallow that, at times, it is almost indiscernible, but don't panic! The recipient drifts into other spheres of consciousness, which is why it is necessary to ask them to take three deep breaths, at the end of the session, to bring them back. They are often reluctant to leave this space of pure bliss, so give them a little time. Better still, if they have had their feet massaged in their own bed, then all they need do is roll over and drift back into this amazing state of consciousness, emerging in their own time, feeling really great.

Healing occurs when going from a state of discomfort and distress, to one of harmony and ease.

Pleasurable after-effects

It is important to explain to the recipient that any reaction they may have to reflexology is a good reaction. Since reflexology works with, and not against, the manifestations of illness, it sometimes happens that the cycles of the 'dis-ease' have to be completed before the recipient can start feeling better. This may mean that they feel worse after reflexology than they did before, which is why reflexology should be received on a regular basis, instead of just as a once off treatment.

Most people feel really fantastic after a session; they have so much energy that they don't immediately know what to do with themselves! Whenever this happens, it means that a favourable energy shift has taken place in their body, with a corresponding and much-needed change of mind. With such renewed enthusiasm for life, they now have a greater capacity to think, with far more clarity, which makes them more tolerant and reasonable. The accompanying peace of mind allows them to sleep so much better and wake up feeling refreshed. They may even remember their dreams, from which they can gain incredible insight and some additional guidance. By becoming more conscious of their mind, body and spirit, they can now show themselves the respect they deserve and, in the process, gain a deeper 'under-standing' of their soul purpose. They really can then enjoy a much improved quality of life!

Excellent signs of healing

Massaging the feet effectively evacuates the mind and body of old, out-dated belief systems and detrimental habits, so that the way is clear for a fresh start and a much more meaningful approach to life. Although the effects of this cleansing process may initially be a bit disturbing, exhausting or disruptive, once completed, there is a fantastic feeling of liberation and release.

Any of the following are excellent signs that the body is helping itself to better health: *headaches* as everything 'comes to a head', and solutions are found; *high temperatures,* to 'let off steam' and eliminate heated emotions; *increased perspiration,* to flush out old fears, anxiety and concern; *runny eyes,* to unleash unshed tears and wash away any sadness in sight; *cold* or *runny nose,* as a means of clearing past irritations; *skin rashes* or *eruptions,* as irrational, boiling emotions that have 'got under the skin' come to the surface to escape; a more virulent *vaginal discharge* in ladies, as frustrating female issues are dispensed with; *increased urination,* to relieve the body of worked through thoughts and emotions; frequent, easier *defecation* to eliminate the wasteful remnants of life's processes; *temporary diarrhoea,* as unnecessary nonsense and unreasonable pressure are removed; vivid recall of *dreams,* to help comprehend life's ongoing events. Encourage the recipient to drink plenty of purified water after the reflexology massage to assist in the flushing through process and hasten the healing.

Unusual reactions

Natural stimulants evoke natural responses, so it is impossible to cause harm with the light, but firm, movements used in reflexology. However, individuals do continually like to challenge themselves, as a test of their inner strength and resourcefulness, which they do by forcing themselves to deal with the most unexpected, and often perceivably adverse, situations. It's all part of their growth experience.

If memories of truly horrendous times come out during reflexology, the recipient may have what seems like a really alarming reaction. Should this happen, remain calm. Allow yourself to be intuitively guided so that you know what to do next. Remember, reflexology is a non-invasive, natural therapy, and so it can only bring to the fore dormant issues that were already resident in the body. Also remind yourself that a seemingly bad reaction is an excellent sign that the healing process has been well activated.

Most bad reactions come from the subconscious arousal of heart-wrenching emotions, which can cause palpations, hyperventilation or panic, all of which indicate a desperate need for immediate release from a truly horrific memory. Immediately go to the solar plexus reflexes (p. 81) and stay calm. Just keep telling yourself that every reaction is a good reaction. Focus on pacifying the recipient via their feet. It shouldn't take long for the effect to take place; in fact, the recipient usually starts feeling more tranquil almost immediately, but be patient if it does take a little longer. Just keep breathing steadily, and then once the recipient has settled down, continue with the massage. On completion encourage them to drink even more purified water than usual, to flush out the extra toxins. Also suggest that they return, within the next day or two, for further reflexology so that their whole being can continue to be balanced. This is not a common occurrence, but it is better to be aware of it so that you know what to do in the event of it ever happening.

Every body is completely responsible for their own thoughts, actions and reactions

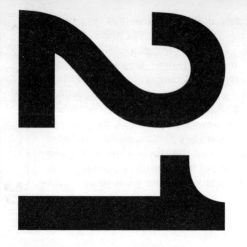

21

preparing for the reflexology massage

In this chapter you will learn:
- how to make the recipient comfortable
- what to tell them
- some handy tips.

Reflexology is a natural healing therapy that is incredibly easy to learn and apply. In fact you already know how to do it because it is an inborn skill that, once rediscovered, can be put to very good use. You are already likely to massage and touch your body in various ways to relieve irritations and different types of discomfort, such as *rubbing* your skin to ease bumps, aching joints or weary muscles, or to stimulate dull, numb areas, or even to get your blood moving and warm your body. You possibly *smear saliva* over insect bites to take away the sting or over cuts to stem minor blood flows. From time to time, you may *scratch* yourself to relieve itching. Then there's the likelihood that you may *stroke*, *pat* or *hug* others, especially when they are upset or grieving, or alternatively to get on their good side!

So it is with reflexology; you will instinctively know exactly what to do, be it stroking, rubbing, tapping and so on! Just allow yourself to be guided intuitively. You can't go wrong, particularly when your intent is good and when you function from the love of your heart. Remember though that whatever you are feeling can have a profound impact on the outcome. Reflexology puts everything back into perspective and makes the difference between having a life and living life to the full. Ready to begin? Let's get started!

Only by venturing into the unknown do you know what you are capable of.

Preparation

Fortunately, you have all that you really need when it comes to doing reflexology, since your hands and your heart are the two most essential items. There are, however, certain standard household goodies that can be used to create a more peaceful and relaxed ambiance, which are best prepared in advance, to ensure a warm and welcoming environment; these include a bed, settee, reclining chair or massage couch with several comfortable pillows and fresh, clean coverings. Also useful are a stool or chair at the foot of the bed for you to sit on; soft music playing gently in the background; beautiful aromas filling the air; flowers or a plant to bring natural energy into the space; a plastic bowl or foot bath, with warm or hot water to soak the feet, plus some recently laundered towels to dry them with afterwards; then some powder, aromatic oils or creams for use during and at the end of the foot massage; and, finally, two glasses filled with purified water.

It's important to create as peaceful a setting as possible, in a subdued environment, so that the recipient can escape the frenetic hustle and bustle of the outside world and relax. It's more a matter of encouraging them to let go visually because, once their eyes are shut, all external impressions dim into oblivion, which is where reflexology steps in to induce inner harmony. The use of a dimmer switch and some softly flickering candle light makes everything in *sight* so much more pleasing, whilst whiffs of aromas from an aromatherapy lamp or incense appeasing the sense of *smell* (see Appendix I). Soothing music creates a *sound* atmosphere (see Appendix III), and the placing of a 'Do not disturb' notice on the door, plus activating a telephone answering machine or service, avoids having to lose *touch* with the recipient. Also, be aware of the furnishings in the room, since pastel colours are subconsciously soothing, whilst bright colours stimulate and can even heighten volatile feelings.

Deep healing requires a willingness and commitment to go deep within.

Communication

If the recipient knows very little about reflexology, or has never had a session, then it's advisable to give them a simple and clear explanation to reassure and relax them. Just knowing that foot massage is a trustworthy and natural process will help them to let go without the fear of being hurt. Tell them what reflexology is, how it works, what to expect during and after the massage, why they may react the way that they do and why it is advisable for them to drink plenty of purified water after the massage so that they then know more or less what to expect.

Those on prescribed medication should let their specialist know that they are planning to have reflexology, so that appropriate adjustments can be made to the dosage, since immediate improvements are likely once the healing process has been activated. The best time for these individuals to receive reflexology is just over an hour before their next medication is due because this is when the drugs are least effective, which makes their body more vulnerable and, therefore, most receptive. Once you have finished explaining everything, invite the recipient to soak their bare feet in the foot spa or plastic bowl for as long as you feel is necessary.

Comfort

When soaking the recipient's feet in the foot bath, make sure that the water is pleasantly warm in winter and refreshingly cool in summer. Consider adding a sprig of lavender or a drop of its oil to relax the recipient and, when it's particularly warm, put in a droplet of peppermint oil since it has a deliciously cooling effect. This is an ideal time to chat and find out more about the recipient, whilst giving them the opportunity to gain confidence in you. Then hand them a fresh towel to dry their feet, or do this for them, after which, you can invite them to lie as flat as possible on the bed or couch.

Make them comfy, with one pillow beneath their head and another one or two pillows under their knees and lower legs, so that their spine is as flat as it can be. Cover them with a light sheet when it's hot and a warm blanket or duvet when it's cold, since body heat is generally lost as they let go. Also for modesty reasons, especially when ladies wear skirts or dresses, since their legs do need to be slightly apart in order to gain sufficient access to all aspects of both feet.

Shake some powder into your hand, rub your palms together, and then spread it gently over both feet, going in between their toes, as a means of facilitating the massage. This also helps the recipient to feel less self-conscious, especially if they have smelly feet due to extreme anxiety. Discourage any further conversation so that they can now drift off into the tranquil alpha state of consciousness and reconnect with their inner self. You are now ready to start the hands on massage with the warm-up technique (p. 152).

Treat everybody as the most important person in the world.

Helpful reminder

Although it is extremely rewarding to see such amazing results so quickly, remember that, when giving reflexology, you are only a conduit, who has taken on the role of encouraging the recipient to relax and be more open to receiving universal energies, so that they can fully utilize these life forces to heal themselves. There is, after all, only one person you can heal and that is yourself!

Rule of thumb

Whether you are giving reflexology to maintain good health or to help somebody feel so much better about themselves, always do a complete foot massage, from top to bottom. Pay particular attention to their nervous system and solar plexus reflexes, also to their endocrine gland and sensory reflexes, as well as to those reflexes that feel distressed. Reflexology is a neutral energy that allows whatever needs to happen, happen!

When you first make contact with your recipient, be conscious of what you are doing because it sets the tone for the whole session. When sequences involve moving from foot to foot, keep going from the right foot to the left foot, although, you will find that most of the massage is done on both feet simultaneously.

22

reflexology step by step

In this chapter you will learn:
- the whole technique
- useful tips
- what to expect.

The warm-up

Start the reflexology session by encouraging the recipient to relax as much as possible through the caressing movements of the warm-up. This is a perfect opportunity to really connect with one another and to gauge what challenges the recipient is facing in their life. Feel free to adapt any of the following techniques to suit their individual needs, as you persuade the recipient to loosen up, so that they are more open to receiving universal energies.

Step 1 – create trust

Take time to establish a bond between you and the recipient because they may be feeling slightly vulnerable, having bared their soles and their soul to you. So start by gently taking the recipient's heels and resting them lightly in the palms of your hands, either with their feet still covered or uncovered. As you do this, invite them to close their eyes and take in three deep breaths (figure 97).

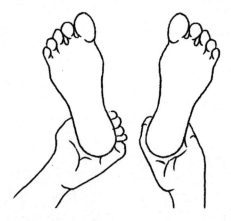

figure 97 rest their feet in your hands

Step 2 – breathe and relax

Guide them as they take these three long, deep breaths and encourage them to hold each breath for as long as possible. As they breathe in, suggest that they take in 'pure love' and 'white light', and, as they breathe out, invite them to let go of anything that no longer needs to be part of them. As they do this, be aware of your own breathing, using it to consciously relax your own body, whilst sending the energy to any tense areas, such as your neck, shoulders, back and upper arms.

Now that you are both much more relaxed, remind the recipient to breathe naturally, as they keep their eyes closed and focus inwards. Meanwhile, keeping your hands as they are, clear your own mind and connect with the compassion coming from your heart. Take time to tune into their energy and listen to what their body is saying. Forget about trying to please and just be your wonderful self! Make up your mind to really enjoy every second of however long the session may take. Remember to vary your pressure throughout the massage, from being really gentle but firm, for physical ease, to barely touching their skin's surface, to help lift their spirit. If you feel that you are highly sensitive to other people's energies, then encase yourself, and the recipient, in a beautiful white or pink bubble, so that you can each enjoy your own space. Then trust your intuition to guide you every step of the way. It's now time for the two of you to experience complete serenity, inner peace and a tremendous boost of life force energy.

You have brought a special gift to this planet – your uniqueness.

Step 3 – caress the tops

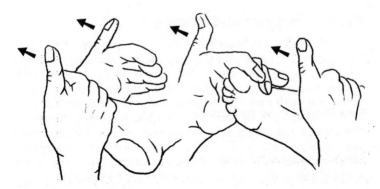

figure 98 caress the tops

Gently lower the recipient's heels onto the bed, then lightly but reassuringly stroke the tops of their feet, hand over hand, towards yourself (figure 98), first on their right foot, then on their left. This is one of the few times that the movements are intentionally towards, and not away from you, because it gives the recipient time to get used to your presence.

Step 4 – stroke their soles

Next stroke the soles of their right foot, and then of their left foot, with the backs of your hands (figure 99), this time towards the recipient, giving them a little longer to feel comfortable with putting themselves in such a vulnerable position.

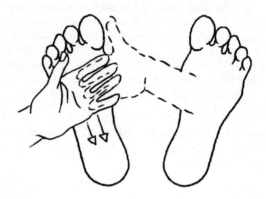

figure 99 stroke their soles

Step 5 – explore and release

Now place all your fingertips, side by side, on top of the right toes (figure 100) and with tiny circular movements, gently ease your fingers over the top of the right foot, up to their ankle crease; then separate your finger tips and continue massaging with these small round movements along either side of their right ankle, to the back of their heels. Repeat the whole procedure three times, reducing your pressure each time, before doing the same on their left foot. This is a great way of easing back tension, which is usually a result of unpleasantness going on in the background of the recipient's life and holding them back.

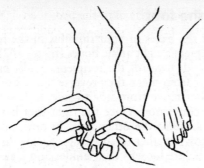

figure 100 explore and release

Step 6 – circle the ankle bones

With your left fingers resting on the outer right ankle bone, and your right fingers on the inner right ankle bone, simultaneously circle around these bones, firmly yet sensitively (figure 101), gradually easing your pressure until there is very little or no contact, whilst, at the same time, steadily removing all your fingers, except your middle fingers, so that, eventually, they are the only ones doing the circling. Now repeat on the left foot. This circling is great for loosening the hip bones. It also reassures the individual that they are in safe hands and encourages them to believe more in themselves.

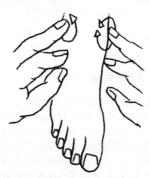

figure 101 circle the ankle bones

Step 7 – shake the foot

Rest the mounds, at the bases of your thumbs, in the hollows either side of the recipient's right ankle bones (figure 102). Now move one of your hands towards the recipient, whilst bringing your other hand away from them; then reverse this action. In so doing, watch their foot move from side to side, at first slowly, and then with more conviction. Once the right foot has had a good shake, do the same to the other foot. In time, and with practice, you will know whether to speed up or slow down the movement. This procedure loosens their ankles and makes it so much easier for the recipient to adapt to life's ups and downs, making them far more flexible and forgiving within their relationships. It also eases the strain of being held back, which gives them the confidence to really step out and make incredible progress.

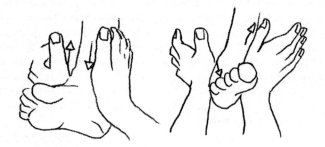

figure 102 shake the feet

Step 8 – pull the Achilles

For the Achilles pull, the recipient must be lying as flat as possible because it's not so effective if they are either sitting up or in any other position. Place your left hand under their right heel, with your right hand aligned on top of the same foot; now gently but firmly 'pull' their right heel towards you (figure 103) until a slight resistance is felt, whilst, at the same time, looking at their body to see it lengthen. Hold the stretch for a while before very slowly releasing. Repeat this three times before doing the same on their left foot. Not only does this give their legs a good stretch, but it also elongates the spine, which releases tension and any trapped nerves. It also helps the spine to realign itself, which, in turn, encourages the free flow of vital life force energies.

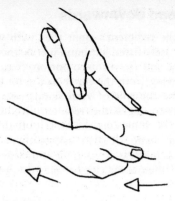

figure 103 pull the Achilles

Step 9 – stretch the Archilles

Take the recipient's right heel back into your left hand, and place your right hand, once again, in alignment on the top. Now gently, but firmly, bend their foot downwards (figure 104), extending the upper surface as far as possible without any resistance. Hold this stretch for a while before allowing the foot to slowly return to its natural position. Repeat three times and then do the same on the other foot. This movement can be alternated with the Achilles pull. Its purpose is to create greater awareness of when to hold back and when to step out front, whilst remaining open to the possibility of being stretched from time to time.

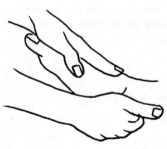

figure 104 stretch the foot

Step 10 – knead downwards

Gently support the recipient's right toes with your right hand and place your loosely fisted left hand just below their toe necks. Knuckle down the sole from top to bottom (figure 105) in long, steady strips, moving from the outer to the inner edges of their right foot. Reverse the role of your hands and repeat on their left foot. This encourages the recipient to literally 'knuckle down' and get on with making the most of their life, by dealing with the tasks in hand. It also assists them in confronting everything they encounter, by opening and clearing their energy pathways, so that their ideas can be put into practice.

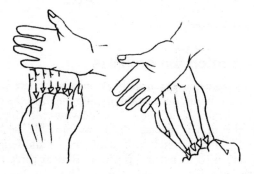

figure 105 knead downwards

Step 11 – rub the spinal reflexes

Using the heel of your right hand caress their bony right arch (figure 106), moving from their big toe to their ankle bone, whilst applying slight pressure on the way up, but then slowly and gently drag your hand back again. Repeat this a few times, before doing the same on their left arch, but, this time, use the heel of your left hand. This is an excellent way of calming the nerves, getting rid of inappropriate beliefs and encouraging complete relaxation.

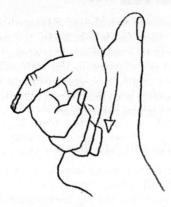

figure 106 rub the spinal reflexes

In between sequences

In between each sequence, massage each foot thoroughly, from top to bottom, to enhance the overall effect of the individual procedures. Start by cupping your hands around their right foot, fingers on top and thumbs underneath, and then move your hands, simultaneously, from the toes to the ankles, where you then separate your hands so that they can continue along either side of the heels (figure 107). Do this at least three times before repeating it on the left foot, to create overall harmony, accelerate the healing process and reassure the recipient. It's also a very effective way of warming cold feet.

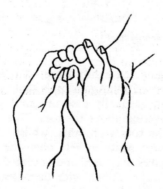

figure 107 in between sequences

Soothe the nerves

The nervous system reflexes are always massaged first because with the brain controlling the whole body, the mind can be calmed and the recipient relieved of any fear or anxiety, thereby allowing their body to relax. By balancing the intellect and the intuition, the recipient can also gain greater insight into what it is that they should be doing with their life so that they can enjoy a more meaningful and manageable journey.

Step 12 – open the energy flows

Begin by opening the energy flows which, in turn, opens the mind. Gently place all your fingertips on top of the corresponding toes, except for the big toes (figure 108). Apply gentle pressure, hold for a few seconds, and then gradually ease off until your fingertips just rest on or hover above the toe surfaces.

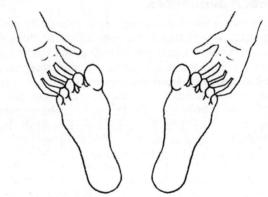

figure 108 open the energy flow 1

Remove your fingers and lightly place your thumb tips on top of the big toes (figure 109). Again apply slight pressure for a few seconds, and then gradually ease off until your thumbs are resting or just hovering above the toes. To enhance the effect, mentally infuse the toes with ether, whilst visualizing indigo, violet, purple and/or white to help open the energy flows up even more. This gives over-used and outdated belief system the opportunity to escape, taking with them fearful notions and frightful memories. The body often jerks and twitches as energy reaches parts that it hasn't been able to access for some time. You may feel tingling or intense warmth between your fingers and the recipient's toes, as you both become increasingly revitalized. This is a truly amazing way of reconnecting with the Universal energies. It encourages the recipient to link with their true spirit so that they can attain greater compassion for themselves, as well as for the whole of humanity. After all, at soul level, we are 'All One'.

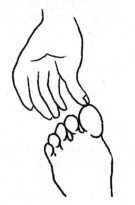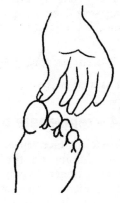

figure 109 open the energy flow 2

Step 13 – ease the mind

Rest either your thumbs or, preferably your little fingers, on the outer edges of the recipient's little toes (figure 110). Gently push down on them for a few seconds, then, as you release, lightly rotate the tips (p. 137). Move your fingers fractionally along the toe tips and repeat this movement, continuing until the tops of both little toes have been well stimulated. Now place your fourth fingers on the outer edges of the fourth toes and repeat; then do the same with your third fingers on the third toes, followed by your second fingers on the second toes and finally your thumbs on the big toes. Return your little fingers to the outer edges of the little toes but, this time, place them slightly lower down; now continue the technique. Keep massaging in strips, across all toe pads, starting a fraction lower down each time changing fingers, until all toe pads have been thoroughly massaged. This helps to take weight off the mind and makes space for exciting new concepts, whilst at the same time assists in improving brain activity. It also expands the capacity to think, calms or excites the hypothalamus, prolongs concentration and alters thought patterns. Ultimately it ensures a much healthier state of mind.

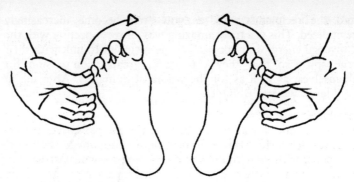

figure 110 ease the mind

Step 14 – rejuvenate the face

To rejuvenate the face repeat the above sequence but this time, place your thumbs on the recipient's toe pads, with your corresponding finger directly opposite, on top of their toes to substantially increase the energy flow. If the vibration is too intense for them, lift your supporting fingers whilst maintaining contact with your thumbs only. Once all the toe pads have been thoroughly massaged (figure 111) milk them all (p. 138) , from the outside to the inside edges of each toe; now feather caress them (p. 139), one by one, from top to bottom, first on their right foot, progressing from the little toe pad to the big toe pad, before repeating on the left toe pads. Remember to spend extra time on 'congested' reflexes and to massage the big toes particularly well since these contain the main brain and sensory reflexes. These movements boost self-confidence and make it so much easier to face the world as an individual.

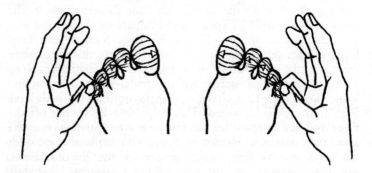

figure 111 rejuvenate the face

Step 15 – improve the eyesight

Place your thumbs over the centres of both little toe pads, with your little fingers directly opposite, on top (figure 112). Lightly squeeze the two digits together until a slight resistance is felt. Hold for a few seconds before gently and slowly rotating your thumbs, whilst, at the same time, visualizing red. Then gradually ease off until there is little or no contact. Now lightly rest your little fingers on the hubs of the toe pads, over the eye reflexes, for a short while. Repeat on the mounds of the fourth toe pads, with your thumbs and ring fingers, whilst visualizing orange; then on the middle of the third toes, with your thumbs and middle fingers, with yellow in mind; on the centres of the second toes with your thumbs and index fingers, picturing green and, finally, on the midpoints of the big toe pads, with your thumbs on the bottom and your second fingers on top, imagining purple and blue. This technique is ideal for improving eyesight, sharpening vision, easing eye strain, broadening the outlook, clarifying perceptions, helping to focus better, maximizing optical functioning and balancing the recipient's interpretation of their emotional environment.

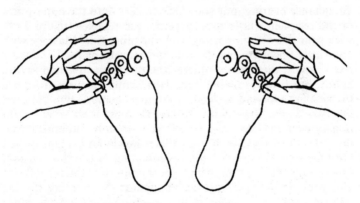

figure 112 improve the eyesight

Step 16 – acknowledge the nose

Acknowledge the nose to make sure that the recipient is on track and doing what they should be doing. This massage helps them find their way by 'following their nose'. Place your thumbs on the inner joints of both big toes (figure 113), with your third fingers providing support on the opposite side. Gradually press in, rotate gently and then release. Now rest the tips of your third fingers on these reflexes for a few seconds, visualizing yellow to enhance the sense of smell and encourage self-recognition.

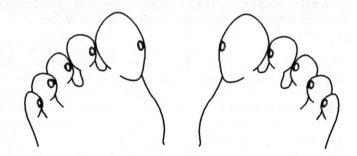

figure 113 acknowledge the nose

Step 17 – for better hearing

To enhance hearing, put your little fingers onto the outer joints of the recipient's little toes, over the ear reflexes (figure 114), with your thumbs supporting from the other side. Massage with your little fingers, using the rotation movement (p. 137), for a few seconds; then gently squeeze the two digits together before lightly, but firmly, milking both sides simultaneously, from top to bottom, applying a slight amount of compression between the two digits. Repeat on the fourth toes, with your fourth fingers over the ear reflexes and your thumbs supporting; go onto the third toes, with your third fingers and thumbs; then onto the second toes, with your second fingers and thumbs and, finally, onto the big toes, with your thumbs over the ear reflexes and your third fingers providing support. Stimulating the ear reflexes improves listening skills, creates awareness of the inner mind chatter, enhances the clarity of sounds and clarifies their meaning, whilst it also increases alertness, improves balance and assists in the accurate interpretation of all that is heard.

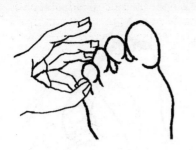
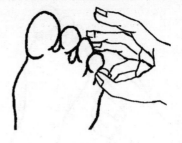

figure 114 for better hearing

Step 18 – soothe the mouth

Place your thumbs onto the mouth reflexes (figure 115) just below the inner joints of both big toes, then using your fourth fingers on the opposite side for support, gradually press in, rotate gently and slowly release. Now place the tips of your fourth fingers on both mouth reflexes for a few seconds, visualizing orange, to facilitate speech, ease decision making, enhance self confidence and for greater belief in personal concepts.

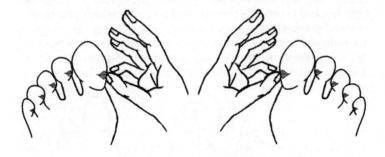

figure 115 soothe the mouth

Step 19 – relax the jaw

Massage the jaw reflexes (figure 116) to ease tension and increase mobility in this area, prevent the grinding of teeth and to increase confidence so that innovative ideas are shared with conviction.

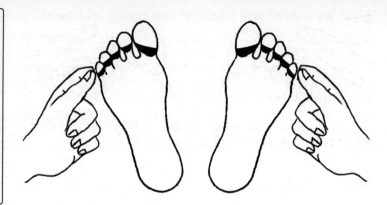

figure 116 relax the jaw

Step 20 – milk the facial lymphatics

To milk the facial lymphatics, place your thumb pads, side by side on top of the right little toe (figure 117) then soothingly, yet firmly, stroke downwards, thumb over thumb, in tiny movements, from top to bottom, several times until the right little toe pad is thoroughly milked. Now do the same on the fourth right toe, followed by the third right toe, then the second right toe and eventually the big right toe, after which you repeat, in exactly the same way, on the left toes. Doing this helps to open the recipient's mind to every point of view by removing mental congestion and deeply ingrained impressions. In so doing, it clears away the old to make way for the new.

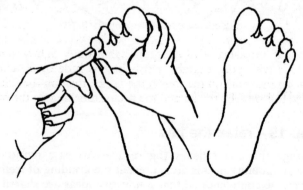

figure 117 milk the facial lymphatics

Step 21 – over the back of the head and neck

To massage the back of the head and neck, place all your fingers either side of the recipient's feet, on the outer edges of their little toes, then move them in unison to 'walk' them over the tops of all the toes (figure 118), finishing on the inner edges of both big toes. Repeat a few times to clear the clutter at the back of the mind and to evacuate fearful memories from the deep subconscious. It also helps strengthen belief in themselves, whilst providing a firm backing for their own ideas.

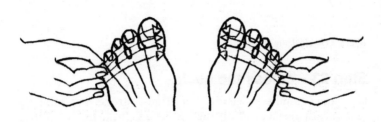

figure 118 over the back of the head and neck

Open the avenues of expression

Step 22 – clear the throat

Put your thumbs onto the recipient's little toe necks, with your third fingers placed directly opposite (figure 119). Gently squeeze the two digits together, hold for a while before gradually releasing whilst, at the same time, lightly rotating (p. 137) with your thumbs, until there is little or no contact. Now do the same on the fourth toe necks, then on the third toe necks, followed by the second toe necks, finishing on the big toe necks.

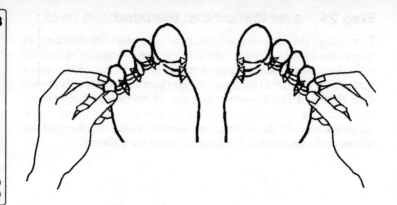

figure 119 clear the throat

Step 23 – caress the neck

Use your thumbs to gently, but firmly, stroke and milk the underneath surfaces of all the toe necks, from top to bottom (figure 120), first on the right toe neck, going from the little to the big toe necks, then do the same on the left toe necks. Give additional attention to the sides, since this is often where there is the most tension, accompanied by a pile of unresolved emotions. Now feather each toe neck, in the same way. This sequence eases neck and throat tension, assists with lymphatic activity and increases blood flow to and from the head, which effectively opens up all the main avenues of self expression.

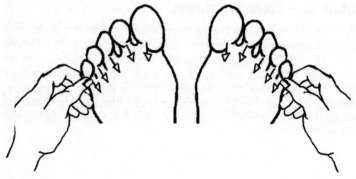

figure 120 caress the neck

Step 24 – a weight off the shoulders

To massage the shoulder reflexes, place your thumbs on the outer edges of the balls of both feet, immediately below the recipient's little toes necks, with your third fingers on top (figure 121). Lightly squeeze the two together then gently rotate (p. 137) with your thumbs as you ease the pressure. Move the digits to beneath the fourth toe necks and repeat the movement. Keep doing this as far as the bases of the second toes. Repeat several times, especially if these reflexes feel hard and swollen or lack substance.

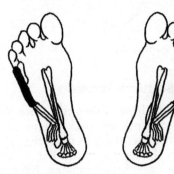

figure 121 ease the load

Step 25 – ease the load

Milk the shoulder reflexes by sliding your thumbs firmly, but gently, around the bases of the little toe necks (figure 122) before slipping them through the gaps between the little and fourth toes; bring your thumbs back again, then slide them around the bases of the fourth toe necks before slipping them through the gaps between the fourth and third toes. Keep doing this as far as the gaps between the second and big toes. Repeat as many times as needed to take a 'weight off the shoulders', to ease the need to 'shoulder responsibilities' and to enhance the flow of life force energies to the head, specifically to the ears and eyes. It also relaxes the clavicle bones, expands the chest and improves stature.

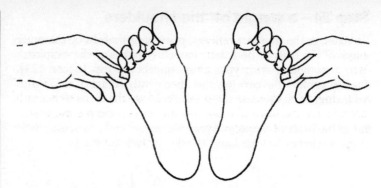

figure 122 a weight off the shoulders

Step 26 – release neck tension

To release tension at the back of the neck, place all your fingers either side of the recipient's toe necks (figure 123) and then 'walk' them, in unison, over the tops of all the toe necks, as far as the inner edges of the big toe necks. Repeat this movement another two to three times before milking. Now lightly run all your fingers, from the tips of the toes, over the tops of the feet, to the ankle creases. All in all, these caresses help to increase neck flexibility so that there is greater harmony between the recipient's internal and external environments.

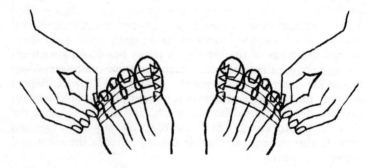

figure 123 release neck tension

Step 27 – balance the mind

Lightly place your third fingers onto the tips of both little toes (figure 124), resting them there for a few seconds before moving onto the joints of your the toes; stay there a while, and now place them at the bases of both little toes. Repeat these three balancing techniques on top of the fourth toes, third toes, second toes and lastly the big toes to help centre the mind and put everything into perspective.

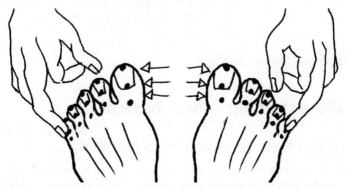

figure 124 balance the mind

Step 28 – stroke the back of the neck and shoulders

Gently caress the tops of both feet by lightly running the tips of all your fingers from the toe nails to the ankles (figure 125) to soothe the anxiety of 'getting it in the neck' or of feeling obliged to take on more than is really necessary. Stroke both feet a few times, from the toes to the ankles, to clear anything hurtful or upsetting that is going on in the background.

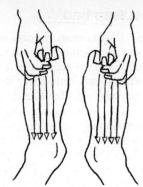

figure 125 soothing the nerves

Re-establish a firm backbone

Step 29 – co-ordinate mind and body

To co-ordinate the mind and body, place your thumbs or fingers on the tips of both big toes (figure 126) and gently massage down the inner edges, as far as their joints, along the recipient's midbrain reflexes. Repeat by moving the digit a fraction either way of the strip, to make sure that the small area is thoroughly massaged. Now milk with tiny soothing strokes and then lightly feather. Doing this fine-tunes muscular co-ordination, improves respiration, enhances cardiac and circulatory functioning and encourages a more balanced approach to life.

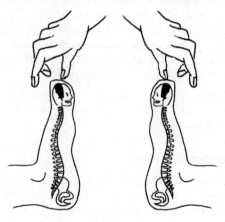

figure 126 co-ordinate mind and body

Step 30 – ensure a firm backing

To strengthen the spine, place your thumbs or fingers on the inner joints of both big toes (figure 127) and gently massage, with rotation or caterpillar movements, along the complete length of the bony ridges that border the insides of the recipient's feet, finishing just beneath the inner ankle bones. Repeat, but this time have your thumbs angled downwards, onto the tops of the bony ridges, to stimulate or calm the sensory nerves. Now do this again, but with your thumbs gently pushing upwards, underneath the bony ridges, to access the motor nerves. Follow by milking first the right spinal reflex, with small, repetitive soothing strokes, from the big toe to the ankle, and then on the left reflex. Finish with an exceptionally light feathering also from top to bottom, which either soothes agitated nerves or stimulates petrified nerves. All the cells benefit from these caresses because all the nerves stem from the spinal cord to infiltrate the whole body. Massaging the spinal reflexes facilitates the relay of nervous messages, whilst, at the same time, increasing each cell's awareness of its environment, enabling it to function at its best.

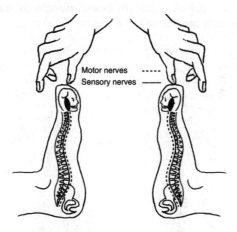

figure 127 ensure a firm backing

Step 31 – ease the neck

Repeat step 30 from the joints of the big toes to their bases (figure 128), especially for neck problems, to increase flexibility so that every point of view can be clearly seen.

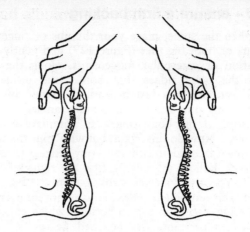

figure 128 ease the neck

Step 32 – caress the upper back

Repeat step 30, along the inner edges of both balls of the recipient's feet (figure 129), to boost emotional backing and support through greater inner strength.

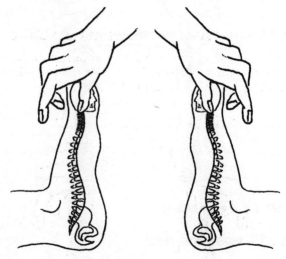

figure 129 caress the upper back

Step 33 – strengthen the upper middle back massage

Repeat step 30, from the bases of both balls of the feet to the waistlines of the feet (figure 130), to provide the strength to keep going no matter what!

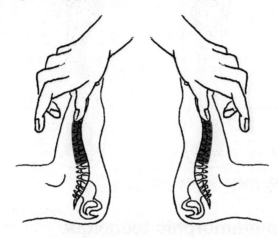

figure 130 strengthen the upper middle back

Step 34 – reassure the lower middle back

Repeat step 30, from the waistline of both feet to the junction of the insteps and heels (figure 131), for enhanced relationships and greater back-up in all forms of communication.

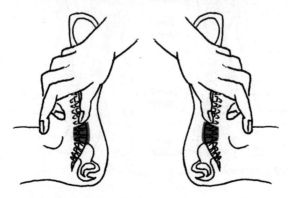

figure 131 reassure the lower middle back

Step 35 – empower the lower back

Repeat step 30, around the bases of the inner ankles (figure 132), to ease lower back pain through self-empowerment and greater inner resourcefulness.

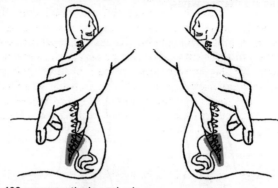

figure 132 empower the lower back

The metamorphic technique

Complete this section of the procedure with the metamorphic technique, which liberates past fears and anxieties, especially those experienced whilst in the womb. The tips of your big toes signify your conception, your spinal reflexes reflect your time in the womb, whilst the ends of the bony ridges, just beneath your inner ankles, represent the time of your birth (figure 133).

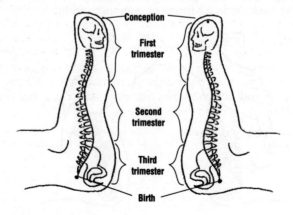

figure 133 reflections of time in the womb

Step 36 – release the past

Lightly place the tips of your third fingers on top of the big toes, which represent the time of conception, and visualize a beautiful white light. Keep your fingers still for a few seconds then, barely touching the skin's surface, glide them slowly over the spinal reflexes, to just beneath the inner ankles, which symbolize the time of birth. Leave your fingers here for a while and, again, visualize a bright white light. Repeat the whole sequence another two to three times. For one or two of the sequences, try using tiny circular movements, instead of just gliding. This powerful technique effectively cuts the invisible umbilical cord between the recipient and their mother. It frees them of the need to be so caught up in each other's energy and allows them to be their own unique individual.

The solar plexus technique

The solar plexus reflexes are the most powerful on the feet and can be massaged at any time to calm the client, should they be panicking for any reason.

Step 37 – create a centre of calm

Place both thumbs on the hollows (figure 134) immediately below the balls of the recipient's feet and apply a gentle, but firm, pressure until a slight resistance is felt. Keep your thumbs still for a while and then gradually ease off, until the tips of your thumbs barely touch the skin's surface. Lightly stroke the reflexes either with your thumbs or third fingers, before resting the tips of your third fingers on the hollows for a few seconds. This immediately creates an inner calm. It also relieves asthmatic attacks and bronchial spasms, soothes palpitations, reduces hysteria and regulates hyperventilation. Massaging these reflexes induces an incredible sense of serenity and peace throughout.

You are what you think!

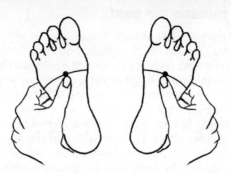

figure 134 create a centre of calm

Harmonize the endocrine system

The endocrine reflexes are generally quite sensitive, especially when there is a related issue. They are always massaged after the nervous system reflexes since they rely on the hypothalamus, at the base of the brain, as well as the nerves, to provide them with the information they need so that they know what to do.

Step 38 – open the energy flow

Start by opening the energy flows (figure 135a and b), as explained in step 12, to make all the glands more receptive to receiving universal input.

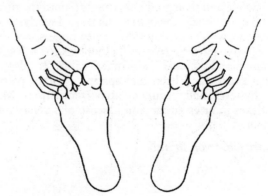

figure 135a open the energy flow

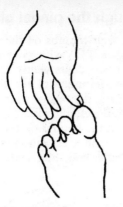
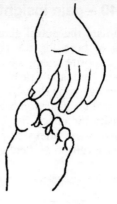

figure 135b opening the energy flow

Step 39 – put the pituitary gland in control

To help the pituitary gland function properly, lightly place your thumbs onto the inner joints of both big toes (figure 136) and apply gentle pressure, whilst gyrating your thumbs at the same time. Hold them still for a while and then gradually ease off. Replace your thumbs with the tips of your third fingers and rest these lightly on the pituitary gland reflexes for a few seconds, whilst visualizing violet for greater clarity. This also calms the emotions, creates inner harmony and balances the hormonal secretions by improving the overall functioning of all endocrine glands.

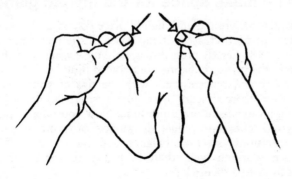

figure 136 put the pituitary gland in control

Step 40 – gain insight through the pineal gland

To stimulate the pineal gland, put your thumbs on the central mounds of both big toe pads (figure 137) with your second fingers opposite them; squeeze the two digits gently together, and then gradually release, whilst rotating with the thumbs. Now remove your thumbs. Lightly rest the tips of your second fingers in their place, on these eye reflexes, and visualise indigo to intensify the effect of harmonizing the natural cycles. It also naturalizes the menstrual cycle, stabilizes mood swings, enhances intuition and enlightens mind, body and soul.

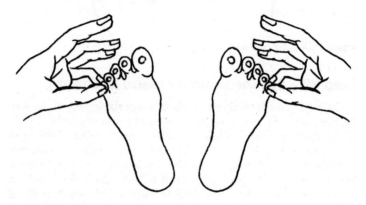

figure 137 gain insight through the pineal gland

Step 41 – make space for the thyroid gland

To massage the thyroid gland, lightly place your thumbs on the inner edges of both creases, at the bases of the recipient's big toes (figure 138). Gently press down, hold for a while, and then, as you ease the pressure, lightly rotate your thumbs. Take your thumbs away and replace them with the tips of your second fingers. Rest these fingers here for a short while, whilst visualizing an exquisite turquoise blue. Now soothingly stroke these thyroid reflexes to reduce the anxiety of trying to get on top of situations, so that balance can be restored. With metabolism working well, there is plenty of space for the recipient to just be themselves.

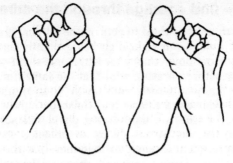

figure 138 make space for the thyroid gland

Step 42 – reconnect with the spirit via the thymus gland

To reconnect with the spirit, use your thumbs to feel for slight indentations or possible swellings, halfway down the inner edges of both balls of the recipient's feet. Keep your thumbs here, whilst placing your index fingers directly opposite (figure 139). Now gently squeeze your digits together and hold for a few seconds. As you ease your pressure, lightly rotate your thumbs. Replace them with your index fingers, which you gently rest on the thymus gland reflexes, whilst visualizing green. Now lightly stroke. This encourages the recipient to really believe in themselves and, in so doing, boost their immunity.

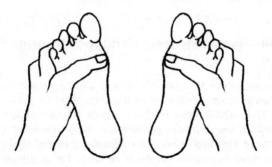

figure 139 reconnect with the spirit via the thymus gland

Step 43 – find courage through the adrenals

Place your thumbs or third fingers on the adrenal gland reflexes (figure 140), with your right digit being slightly further in and fractionally more down than your left. Apply slight pressure and hold briefly before releasing whilst, at the same time, using the rotation technique. Gently milk with your thumbs, feather caress with your third fingers and finish by lightly resting the tips of these fingers on the adrenal gland reflexes for a few seconds. Visualizing yellow helps to enhance the effect by putting the recipient at ease, so that they find the courage to implement their extraordinary and often unbelievable concepts, no matter what others say or think, making the seemingly impossible possible.

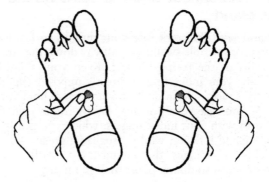

figure 140 find courage through the adrenal glands

Step 44 – generate new concepts through the ovaries

Massage the ovary reflexes on both genders because male and female energies are present in everybody. Start by placing your thumbs or fourth fingers on both ovary reflexes (figure 141), apply slight pressure, hold for a while, then gradually ease off whilst gently rotating with your thumbs. Lightly stroke, then rest your fourth fingers on both reflexes for a few seconds, visualizing orange. Massaging the ovary reflexes enhances the ongoing generation of new concepts, whilst also encouraging the recipient to connect with their gentler, more sensitive feminine energies.

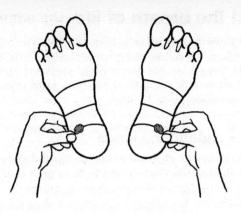

figure 141 generate new concepts through the ovaries

Step 45 – test the way with the testes

You may need to feel around the inner heels, to find the testes reflexes, since they do tend to move. Once you have found them, put your thumbs or little fingers on their reflexes (figure 142), press down slightly, and then, as you ease off, gently massage. Milk lightly with your thumbs, before feathering with your little fingers, visualizing red. This helps to ensure a worthwhile contribution to the advancement of humankind.

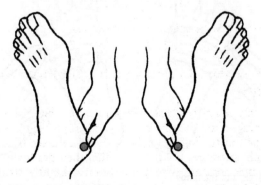

figure 142 test the way with the testes

In between each sequence, massage each foot thoroughly, from top to bottom, to enhance the overall effect of the individual procedures as detailed on p. 159.

Take in the breath of life

The respiratory and cardiac system reflexes are massaged to help individuals become reacquainted with their true spirit through the breath of life. Since these areas are linked to the recipient's self-esteem and self-worth, they assist them in feeling better about themselves and others.

Step 46 – expand the lungs

To expand the lungs, place your thumbs, immediately below the shoulder reflexes, either side of the balls of both feet, with your second fingers on the opposite surface (figure 143). Gently, but firmly, squeeze the two digits together, and then slowly release, whilst lightly rotating with your thumbs. Move both digits fractionally along, and keep doing this until the horizontal strips, across the balls of the feet, have been thoroughly massaged. Return your digits to the outer edges, a fraction lower down, and do the same on the next strip. Continue this, all the way down the balls of both feet, to ensure that there is plenty of space in which to breathe, which then allows the recipient to adapt, more effortlessly, to the constant changes within their emotional environment.

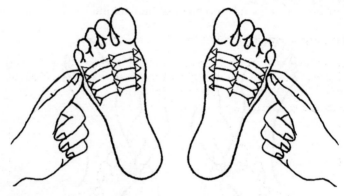

figure 143 expand the lungs

Step 47 – take it all in

Once again, place your thumbs onto the balls of both feet, just below the little toes (figure 144) and then either caterpillar or rotate them downwards in vertical strips, from top to bottom, until the balls of both feet have been completely massaged. Go back to the outer edges of the right foot and this time, milk firmly downwards, thumb over thumb, from the outer to the inner edges. Now, very lightly feather caress with your index fingers. Repeat on the left balls of the feet.

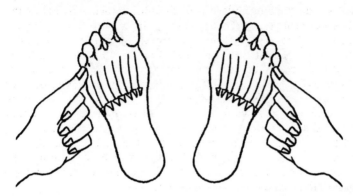

figure 144 take it all in

Step 48 – keep abreast

The breasts are automatically caressed along with the lung reflexes (figure 145). In so doing, emotional congestion is eased, which facilitates the nurturing process and creates more harmonious internal and external environments.

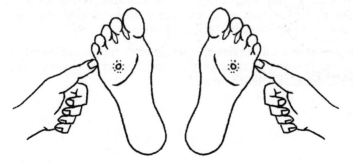

figure 145 keep abreast

Step 49 – renew the love in the heart

To renew the love in the heart, lightly place the tips of your second and third fingers over the heart reflexes (figure 146). Now apply slight pressure for a while, and then gradually ease off gently rotating the digits. Stop for a moment before lovingly stroking these sensitive reflexes, whilst visualizing green or pink to enhance the effect. This movement strengthens and purifies the recipient's affections and opens their heart to greater love for themselves and others. Wherever there's love, there is health.

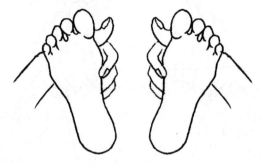

figure 146 renew the love in the heart

Step 50 – firm up the ribcage

To massage the ribcage reflexes, place all your fingers either side of the balls of both feet and 'walk' them in unison over the tops of the recipient's feet (figure 147). Repeat this several times and then, using the heels of your hands, gently caress the upper surfaces, from their toes to their ankles. Finish by lightly running all your fingers over the tops of their feet in the same direction. The idea is to encourage them to find the inner strength to emotionally back themselves.

In between each sequence, massage each foot throughly, from top to bottom, to enhance the overall effect of the individual procedures as detailed on p. 159.

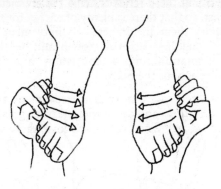

figure 147 firm up the ribcage

Restore the digestive system

There are two parts to your digestive system; your accessory organs, such as your liver, pancreas and spleen, which aid digestion, based on all that happened in the past; and the tract itself, which processes all that is happening now. Massage the former first, to help things settle down, especially if the recipient has just been through a rough patch, so that these organs are in a much better state to help out in the present.

Step 51 – enliven the liver

Stimulate the liver reflexes (figure 148) by placing your left thumb on the outer edge at the top of the right instep, whilst putting your right thumb, a fraction lower, on the opposite edge of the same foot. Either caterpillar or rotate your left thumb, across the top edge of the fleshy instep, from the recipient's right to their left, until it is just above your right thumb. Now remove your left thumb and place it back where it started but, this time, a little lower down than before; and then keep it still. Now massage with your right thumb, from the recipient's left to their right, from the inner to the outer edges of their instep. Continue to alternate your digits, in this way, until the whole triangular reflex of the liver is thoroughly massaged. Now milk firmly downwards, thumb over thumb, followed by a light feathering caress with your third and fourth fingers, from top to bottom. A tiny portion of the liver is also reflected onto the left foot, but since this is massaged at the same time as the left stomach reflex (p. 192), it requires no specific action, unless you feel that it needs it. Massaging these reflexes helps the recipient's liver to sort out the past, so that there is plenty of energy for the present, which then gives them the impetus to implement their own ideas, for their ongoing personal growth and development. It also helps in maintaining a consistent and favourable temperature throughout the body.

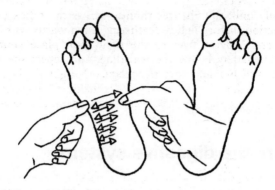

figure 148 enliven the liver

Step 52 – have the gall

When massaging the gall bladder (figure 149), rest your left thumb or third finger on its reflex, midway along the triangular edge of the liver reflex, on the right foot only. Gently rotate your digit, then milk thumb over thumb on the same spot, in a downward movement, before lightly feathering with your third fingers. This helps to dissipate resentment and bitterness, so that the recipient can move on with peace of mind.

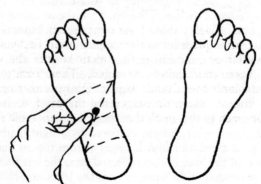

figure 149 have the gall

Step 53 – please the pancreas

To soothe the pancreatic reflexes, place your left thumb immediately below the waistline of the recipient's left foot, and leave it there, to use as a guideline (figure 150). Now place your right thumb on the tip of this tadpole-shaped reflex and caterpillar or rotate it from the recipient's left to their right. Then firmly milk thumb over thumb, across the reflex in the same direction, before lightly feathering downwards with your third fingers. Moving over to the right foot, place your left thumb immediately below the waistline, and repeat the same procedure, still moving from the recipient's right to their left, and going as far as the centre. This helps to balance the pancreas, which means that the recipient can feel at peace about all that is happening around them.

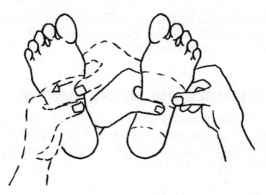

figure 150 please the pancreas

Step 54 – surprise the spleen

With your thumbs either side of the spleen reflex (figure 151), on the upper, outer quadrant of the recipient's left fleshy instep, gently caterpillar or rotate in both directions until the whole reflex has been thoroughly massaged. Then firmly milk downwards, thumb over thumb, before lightly feathering with your third fingers. This encourages the recipient to have a balanced approach to life, in all that they do for themselves and others.

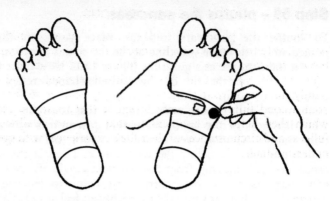

figure 151 surprise the spleen

In between each sequence, massage each foot throughly, from top to bottom, to enhance the overall effect of the individual procedures as detailed on p. 159.

Re-energize the whole system

Start massaging the digestive tract itself from the mouth reflexes, on the big toes, and finish at the anal reflexes, on the inner heels, although the bulk of the digestive organ reflexes are reflected onto the sole insteps

Step 55 – mouth the way

Place your thumbs or fourth fingers on the mouth reflexes (figure 159), just below the joints of the big toes; apply slight pressure and gently rotate to facilitate the chewing process and improve the sense of taste.

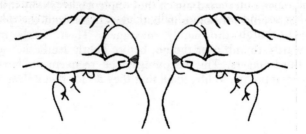

figure 152 mouth the way

Step 56 – soothe the oesophagus

Soothe the oesophagus reflexes by caterpillaring or rotating, with your thumbs or second figures, all the way down, from the mouth reflexes, along the throat reflexes and down the inner edges of the balls of both feet. Do this several times and then lightly milk with your thumbs and gently feather stroke with your second fingers, to pacify or excite the peristaltic action, which then helps the recipient to take in, and swallow, the fullness and circumstances of their life's experiences with greater understanding.

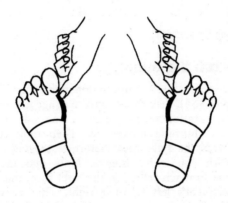

figure 153 soothe the oesophagus

Step 57 – open the stomach

At the entrance of the stomach is the cardiac sphincter, the reflexes of which (figure 154) are massaged to make the stomach more receptive. To do this, rest either your thumbs or second fingers on these reflexes and apply slight pressure; hold for a few seconds, then gradually release, before gently stroking with your thumbs.

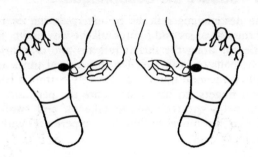

figure 154 open the stomach

Step 58 – rub the tummy

Visualize the stomach reflex in the upper, inner quadrant of the left foot (figure 155), then thoroughly massage it, either with the caterpillar or rotation technique from one side to the other, mimicking its churning movement. Then milk thumb over thumb, towards the right foot, before feathering in the same direction, with your third fingers. Now massage the small portion of the stomach reflex on the right foot, this time going from the recipient's left to their right. This assists them in 'stomaching' all of life's experiences, whilst enhancing their ability to cope, no matter what comes their way.

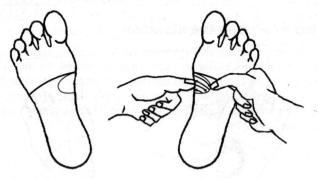

figure 155 rub the tummy

Step 59 – move it on

At the exit of the stomach is the pyloric sphincter, the reflex of which is massaged (figure 156) by applying slight pressure, holding this for a few seconds, then slowly releasing, before lightly massaging with your third fingers. This helps the recipient decide how best to move on to the next stage of their life.

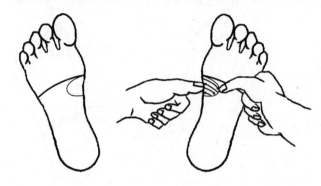

figure 156 move it on

Step 60 – around the 'C' of the duodenum

Use your right thumb to massage the C-shaped duodenum reflex, which is only on the inner, upper quadrant of the right foot (figure 157). As you caterpillar or rotate the 'C' feel free to change thumbs midway, to make the movement flow better; then lightly milk the 'C', before gently feathering. All of this helps the recipient to finish dealing with their past so that they can get on and enjoy their present.

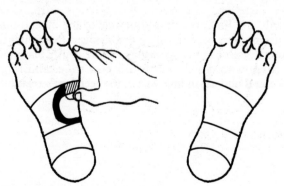

figure 157 around the 'C' of the duodenum

Step 61 – cajole the jejunum

Massage the jejunum reflex (figure 158), which is just above or on the waistline of the left foot, moving from the recipient's right to their left. Then gently milk the reflex, thumb over thumb, in the same direction, before lightly feathering, with your third fingers, to cajole the recipient into taking the next exciting step in the process by keeping things moving.

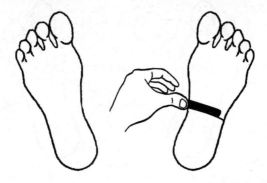

figure 158 cajole the jejunum

Step 62 – wind through the small intestines

Wind through the small intestines by placing your right thumb or fourth finger at the start of the small intestine reflex (figure 159), then massage from the recipient's left to their right, using the base of the waistline, on both feet, as a guideline, as you go from their left to their right foot. Once you have reached the edge of their right foot, return with your left thumb, massaging in the opposite direction, just below the previous strip. Continue, backwards and forwards, from one side to the other, until both lower insteps have been thoroughly massaged. Now lightly milk with your thumbs, in the same way, before gently feathering the whole area with your fourth fingers, to establish greater tolerance and understanding within the recipient's relationships.

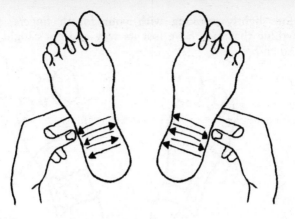

figure 159 wind through the small intestines

Step 63 – reassure the ileo-caecal valve

Place your right thumb or fourth finger on the ileo-caecal valve reflex (figure 160), in the lower, outer corner of the right fleshy instep, and then apply slight pressure (figure 160). Hold this for a while, before gradually releasing, whilst gently rotating. Now lightly stroke the reflex with your fourth fingers, to help get rid of the old and make way for the new.

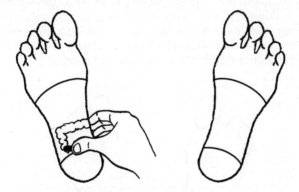

figure 160 reassure the ileo-caecal valve

Step 64 – clear out the appendix

Place your left thumb or fourth finger on the appendix reflex (figure 161), which is only on the recipient's right foot. Then massage this miniscule reflex with tiny rotational movements before lightly stroking with your fourth fingers, to clear anything that may have lost its way and got caught up in a dead end.

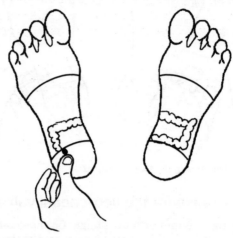

figure 161 clear out the appendix

Step 65 – up the ascending colon

Put your left thumb at the base of the ascending colon reflex (figure 162), and massage up the reflex, as far as the waistline, before milking it firmly with both thumbs, and then lightly feathering with your fourth fingers, to facilitate the ongoing movement of all that remains following what was done or not done, that would otherwise waste time and energy.

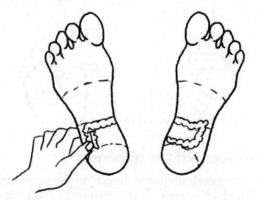

figure 162 up the ascending colon

Step 66 – around the hepatic flexure

Feel for a swelling on or just below the waistline (figure 163) of the right foot. Apply slight pressure, hold it for a while, and then release. Now turn the digit so that it is points towards the left foot. This will assist the recipient in turning corners.

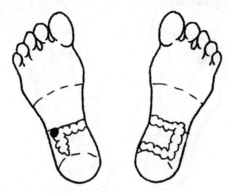

figure 163 around the hepatic flexure

Step 67 – across the transverse colon

Massage the transverse colon reflexes (figure 164), from the recipient's right to their left, following the base of the waistline, first on the right foot, and then on the left. When you get to the centre of the left foot, start massaging slightly upwards, towards the outer edge of the left foot and then firmly milk in the same way, before gently feathering with your fourth fingers. This helps to relieve the pressure of having to perform and meet unreasonably high expectations.

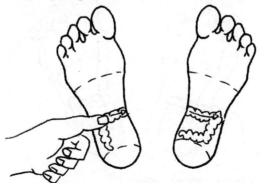

figure 164 across the transverse colon

Step 68 – around the splenic flexure

With your left thumb, feel for the slight swelling of the splenic flexure reflex (figure 165); then massage it well. Now put your right thumb, angled downwards, and apply slight pressure. Hold for a while and then release, to prevent any hiccups getting in the way of progress.

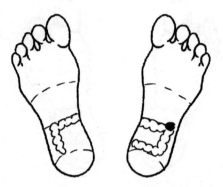

figure 165 around the splenic flexure

Step 69 – down the descending colon

With your right thumb, still pointing downwards, massage down the outer border of the left instep, as far as the heel (figure 166), then firmly milk with both thumbs, before lightly feathering with your fourth fingers, to clear the way along the descending colon.

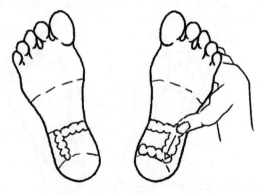

figure 166 down the descending colon

Step 70 – skirt the sigmoid flexure

Rest your right thumb on the sigmoid flexure reflex, in the lower corner of the left sole instep (figure 167), apply slight pressure. Hold for a while, and then release; now turn your thumb so that it is pointing towards the inside edge of the left foot.

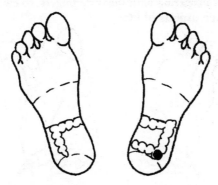

figure 167 skirt the sigmoid flexure

Step 71 – slither along the sigmoid colon

Slither your right thumb along the sigmoid colon reflex, which is along the base of the left instep, from the recipient's left to their right (figure 168); and then firmly milk thumb over thumb, before lightly feathering with your fourth fingers, to keep things moving, especially those things that are on their way out.

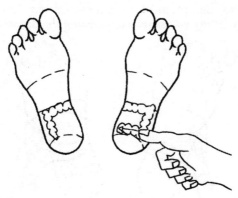

figure 168 slither along the sigmoid colon

Step 72 – out through the rectum

Massage the arcs of the rectum reflexes by placing your thumbs or little fingers on the inner edges of both feet, at the junction of the recipient's heel and instep (figure 169), by either caterpillaring or rotating; then firmly milk thumb over thumb, before gently feathering with the little fingers, to ease the release of all the rough aspects of life.

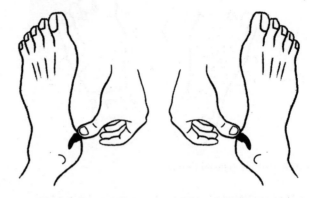

figure 169 out through the rectum

Step 73 – angling for the anus

Apply slight pressure to the anus reflexes (figure 170), hold it for a few seconds, and then release, before firmly stroking the reflexes with your thumbs and caressing with your little fingers. This allows the recipient to experience the utter relief of completely letting go, thereby completing the digestive process.

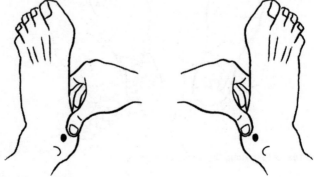

figure 170 angling for the anus

Step 74 – over the middle back

Place all your fingers on the outer edges of both insteps (figure 171) and 'walk' them in unison over the tops, from the outside to the inside. Repeat several times, then lightly run the tips of your fingers, from the base of the toes to the ankle creases, to help provide the inner strength to carry on.

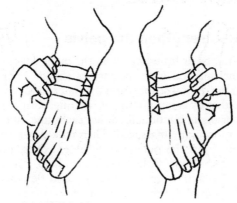

figure 171 over the middle back

Step 75 – soothing the innards

Use all your fingers to walk along the fleshy inner edges of the insteps (figure 172), which can be found immediately beneath the bony arch. Now milk, with the heels of your hands, moving towards the recipient, and then, finally, run all your fingers along these reflexes, to ensure ongoing resourcefulness.

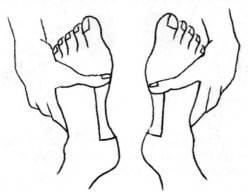

figure 172 soothing the innards

In between each sequence, massage each foot throughly, from top to bottom, to enhance the overall effect of the individual procedures as detailed on p. 159.

Re-instate the bones, muscles and skin

Step 76 – strengthen the pelvis

Put your thumbs or little fingers on the outer edges of both heel pads, at the junction with the insteps (figure 173) and firmly massage in horizontal strips, from the outer to the inner edges of the heels, either by caterpillaring or rotating. Keep repeating this, moving your digits fractionally down each time, until both heels have been thoroughly massaged. Then milk downwards, thumb over thumb, from the outer to the inner edges, before lightly feathering with your little fingers, to help provide a solid foundation, as well as greater mobility and flexibility, which is particularly helpful during childbirth.

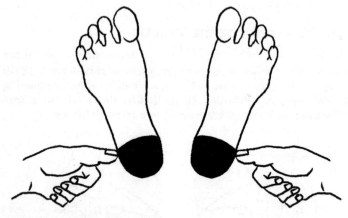

figure 173 strengthen the pelvis

In between each sequence, massage each foot throughly, from top to bottom, to enhance the overall effect of the individual procedures as detailed on p. 159.

Restrengthen the limbs

Step 77 – along the upper arm reflexes

Place your thumbs or your second fingers immediately below your little toes and massage along the outer edges of the balls of both feet (figure 174), to the elbow reflexes. Then firmly milk thumb over thumb and finally feather caress to give the recipient the confidence to reach out and embrace new beginnings.

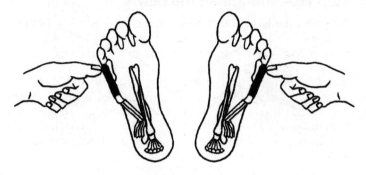

figure 174 along the upper arm reflexes

Step 78 – flex the elbows

Generously use the rotation technique on the elbow reflexes (figure 175), then firmly milk them, before lightly feathering with your second and third fingers, to give the recipient room to be themselves.

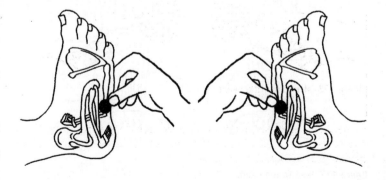

figure 175 flex the elbows

Step 79 – down the lower arm

Use your thumbs, or third fingers, to massage the lower arm reflexes (figure 176), which are between the elbow and hand reflexes along the outside edges of both feet. Then firmly milk along these reflexes, thumb over thumb, before caressing with your third fingers, to help the recipient cope with any challenges they are facing.

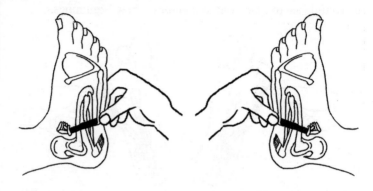

figure 176 down the lower arm

Step 80 – tend to the hands

Tend to the hands (figure 177) in the same way as the elbow reflexes (step 78), to make it easier for the recipient to handle everything that comes their way.

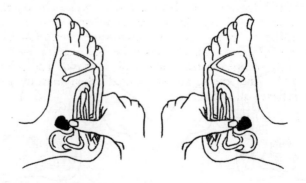

figure 177 tend to the hands

Step 81 – up the thighs

Massage the reflexes for the thighs (figure 178), by placing your thumbs or your fourth fingers on the knee reflexes, then caterpillaring or rotating up towards the base of the outer ankle bones. Now milk with both thumbs, before stroking lightly with your fourth fingers, to help the recipient be more open to moving on.

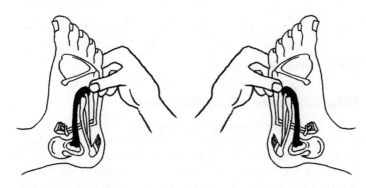

figure 178 up the thighs

Step 82 – knead the knees

Put your thumbs on the recipient's shoulder reflexes and your third fingers on their elbow reflexes, and then use your second fingers to feel for the tiny bony ledges, just above the midway point between the two reflexes. These are the secondary accesses to the knees (figure 179). Now place your thumbs on these reflexes and apply slight pressure, release and massage thoroughly, and then stroke lightly, with your third fingers, to encourage greater flexibility. This helps the recipient to adapt more easily to unexpected changes of direction. The primary reflexes, for the knees, are stimulated when massaging the breast reflexes (p. 185).

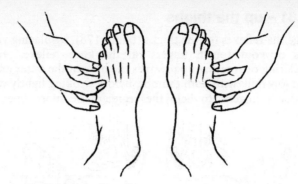

figure 179 knead the knees

Step 83 – skim along the shins

Either caterpillar or rotate your thumbs, or third fingers, along the outer borders of both feet, from the knee to the feet reflexes; then thoroughly milk with your thumbs, before gently feathering with your second fingers. Skim along the shin reflexes (figure 180) to give the recipient greater scope and strength, especially when it comes to following through with their activities.

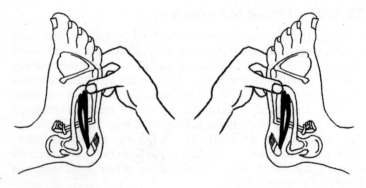

figure 180 skim along the shins

Step 84 – embrace the feet

Massage the foot reflexes (figure 181) by rotating your thumbs, then stroking and feathering to provide even greater stability and mobility.

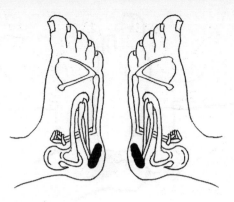

figure 181 embrace the feet

Step 85 – bolster the buttocks

Caress the buttock reflexes (figure 182) on outer triangular areas of both heels either with your thumbs, or all your fingers, several times. Then soothe these areas with the heels of your hands, before lightly feathering with all of your fingers, to help the recipient empower themselves.

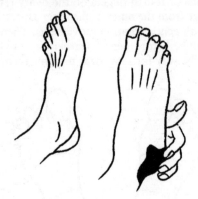

figure 182 bolster the buttocks

Step 86 – reinforce the hips

Circle around the hip reflexes (figure 183) on the outer ankle bones, several times, with either your thumbs, or all your fingers, first firmly, then lightly to provide the impetus and force that the recipient needs to move ahead with ease.

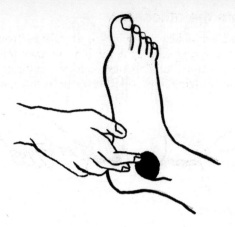

figure 183 reinforce the hips

Appease the reproductive organs

Step 87 – attend to the fallopian tubes

Place your thumbs or fourth fingers on the ovary reflexes (figure 184), and massage from the outer to the inner aspects of the lower fleshy insteps, with gentle rotation movements. Then lightly milk thumb over thumb, before gently feathering with your fourth fingers, to clear the way for new ideas to come through.

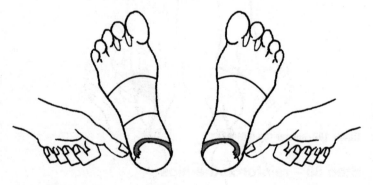

figure 184 attend to the fallopian tubes

Step 88 – from the other side

Now massage the secondary fallopian tube reflexes from the other side this time (figure 185) by caterpillaring, then milking, from the outer to the inner ankle bones, along the ankle creases, to further assist in bringing new concepts out into the open.

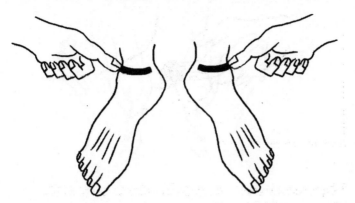

figure 185 from the other side

Step 89 – unleash the uterus

Gently massage the uterus reflexes (figure 186), with your thumbs or little fingers, then lightly stroke and caress them, especially during pregnancy, to create a more harmonious environment within the home, as well as to balance the feminine energy.

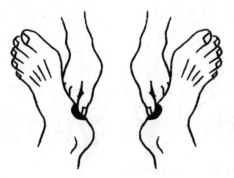

figure 186 unleash the uterus

Step 90 – soothe the vagina

Soothe the vaginal reflexes (figure 187), by rotating either with your thumbs or your little fingers on these slight indentations, then gently stroke and caress them, to encourage a much gentler approach to life.

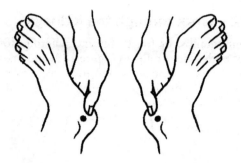

figure 187 soothe the vagina

Step 91 – bolster manly assets

Thoroughly massage the inner triangular areas on both heels, either with your thumbs or with all of your fingers, then milk well, before feathering with your little fingers. Massage the male reproductive reflexes (figure 188) to improve inner strength, enhance personal performance and make the recipient feel important, so that they rise appropriately to any occasion.

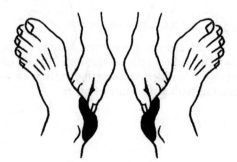

figure 188 bolster manly assets

In between each sequence, massage each foot throughly, from top to bottom, to enhance the overall effect of the individual procedures as detailed on p. 159.

Release the past

Step 92 – work through the kidneys

Place your thumbs, or fourth fingers, pointing downwards, at the top of both kidney reflexes (figure 189) and massage the tiny strips of about an inch, from top to bottom, either by caterpillaring or rotating your digits. Then milk thoroughly with your thumbs, before feathering with your third and fourth fingers, to encourage a harmonious environment and the ideal balance within relationships.

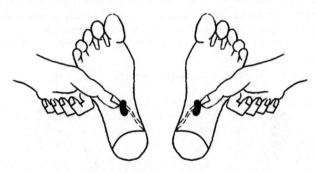

figure 189 work through the kidneys

Step 93 – squeeze the ureters

To milk the ureter reflexes, place your thumbs or fourth fingers midway down the kidney reflexes (figure 190) and caterpillar or rotate down to the bladder reflexes; then milk with your thumbs before feathering with your fourth fingers.

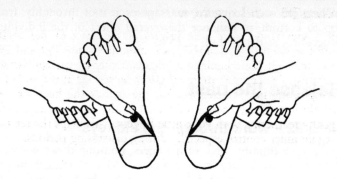

figure 190 squeeze the ureters

Step 94 – reassure the bladder

Place your thumbs or little fingers on the fleshy mounds, at the bases of the inner heels (figure 191) and gently palpate these reflexes, before lightly milking them, and then softly feathering with your little fingers, to make the bladder much more accommodating.

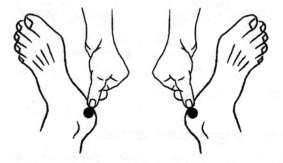

figure 191 reassure the bladder

Step 95 – aid the flow

Put your thumbs or little fingers at the start of the urethra reflexes, on the edges of the fleshy mounds (figure 192 and 193), and massage their significant lengths, either by caterpillaring or rotating. Concentrate on the slight indentations at the end of the females urethra reflexes and on the tips of the heels on male urethral reflexes; then firmly milk with your thumbs, before gently feathering with your little fingers. This helps the recipient regain inner control especially during distressing periods.

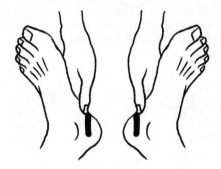

figure 192 aid the flow on females

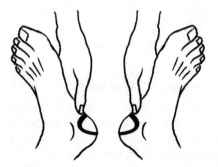

figure 193 aid the flow on males

In between each sequence, massage each foot thoroughly, from top to bottom, to enhance the overall affect of the individual procedures as detailed on p. 159.

The finale

By this time, the recipient should be completely relaxed, making it an ideal opportunity to gently stretch and extend the feet for greater flexibility and expansion of mind, body and soul.

Step 96 – stretch the mind and spine

Gently pull both little toes simultaneously (figure 194), then the fourth toes, followed by third toes, then the second toes, and finally the big toes, giving these large toes a slightly longer pull. This is an excellent way to relieve neck tension, headaches, back disorders, as well as to get the recipient to really open up to all the possibilities that are available to them.

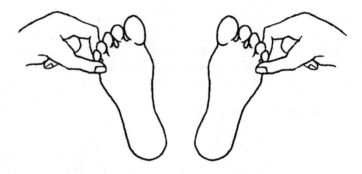

figure 194 stretch the mind and spine

Step 97 – extend the neck

Lightly support the base of the right little toe, with your left thumb and index finger, then, by holding the right little toe between your right thumb and index finger, rotate it, first anti-clockwise and then clockwise (figure 195). Do the same with the fourth right toe, and then each of the other toes, one by one. Now repeat on the left foot, starting with the left little toe and finishing with the left big toe. Spend extra time on rotating both big toes to loosen up the mind and body.

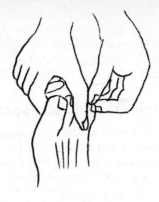

figure 195 extend the neck

Step 98 – flex the upper body

Place your hands either side of the recipient's right foot and gently roll it, side to side (figure 196); then repeat on the left foot. This facilitates the give and take in life, making it easier to expand and contract, which, in turn, boosts the morale.

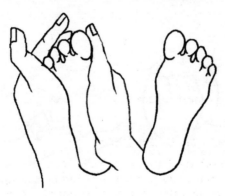

figure 196 flex the upper body

Step 99 – expand the whole being

With both hands on top of the recipient's feet, gently, but firmly, stretch both feet downwards and hold for a while (figure 197a and b). Then place the palms of your hands flat against the soles and coax both feet upwards. This helps broaden the recipient's horizons and encourages a more amenable approach to life.

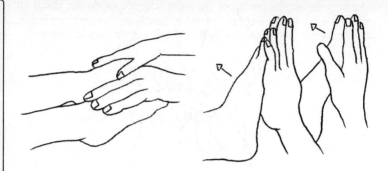

figure 197a and b expand the whole being

Step 100 – relax the lower torso

Support the right heel with your left hand, and use your right hand to rotate the right foot, as widely as possible, first anti-clockwise and then clockwise (figure 198). Change hands and repeat on the left foot, to help balance the odds and keep life events in proportion.

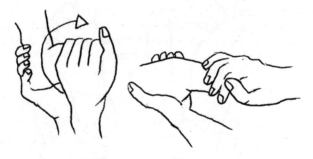

figure 198 relax the lower torso

Step 101 – loosen up

Place your thumbs together, in the middle of the right foot, immediately beneath the toe necks, with your fingers resting on top (figure 199). Then gently push up with your thumbs, whilst using your fingers to lightly stretch the right foot over them. Repeat this several times, as your hands gradually progress all the way down the centre of the right foot. Now do the same on the left foot, to encourage a more relaxed and content approach to life, whilst, at the same time, energizing the whole being.

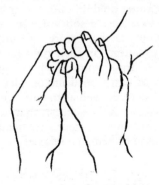

figure 199 loosen up

Step 102 – the final step

Complete the reflexology sequence by massaging the solar plexus reflexes for around a minute. Place your thumbs on the hollows (figure 200), immediately below the balls of the recipient's feet, and apply gentle pressure, until a slight resistance is felt. Then, keep your thumbs still for a while, before slowly easing off, until the tips of your thumbs barely touch the skin's surface. Now lightly stroke the reflexes, either with your thumbs or third fingers, before resting the tips of your third fingers on the hollows for a few seconds.

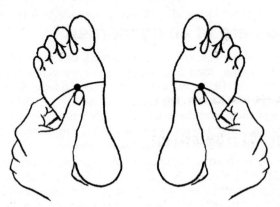

figure 200 the final step

Step 103 – ending the session

Stroke first the right foot, from top to bottom, and then the left foot in the same way. Now cover both feet, with the sheet or blanket, but continue holding onto the covered feet for a little longer. As you do so, use a soft voice to invite the recipient to take in three deep breaths, before opening their eyes, so that they can begin to surface in their own time. Then give them a glass of water to drink immediately, to ground them, whilst reminding them to carry on drinking plenty of water to help flush out their system, as well as to enhance the effect of having their feet massaged. Also suggest that they wrap up well, especially if it's cold outside, since a tremendous amount of heat can be lost, because of being so relaxed.

First-aid reflexology

Ideally always give a complete massage on both feet to ensure overall well-being through homoeostasis of mind, body and soul. Occasionally, however, when there is insufficient time, giving a quick massage is better than nothing. This entails massaging all the toes thoroughly (steps 12–28), soothing the spinal reflexes (steps 29–36), pacifying the solar plexus reflexes (step 37), and balancing the energy centres (steps 38–45), always finishing with the 'in between' massage (p. 159) of both feet. If there is discomfort in a particular part of the body, then massage its related reflex or reflexes as well. End the short massage by soothing the solar plexus reflexes (step 37).

If you are at all concerned

If, at any time, you are at all concerned, or the recipient panics for any reason, then immediately place your thumbs on their solar plexus reflexes and ask them to take in long, deep breaths. Guide them into relaxing more and more on each out breath. Reassure them that the reaction is only temporary and that it is a good sign that a favourable shift has taken place. If available, also give them a few drops of rescue remedy.

23

a summary of the massage

In this chapter you will learn:
- the overall sequence
- about general effects of the foot massage
- about reflexology's role in the future.

The sequence

The following is to assist you in your understanding as to why the feet are massaged in a particular sequence and as a quick reference.

Warm-up

Always begin with the general massage, known as the warm-up (steps 3–11), the caressing movements of the warm-up reassure the recipient that it is okay to relax. They also help to create a trusting relationship between the two of you, whilst giving you the ideal opportunity to pick up on their greatest needs, via their feet.

Sorting out the mind

The brain and sensory reflexes (steps 12–21) are always massaged first, since the whole body is completely dependent upon the recipient's state of mind, which relies on the input from their senses. The soothing movements either calm or stimulate the nerves, balance the intellect and intuition, soothe or excite the emotions, pacify or heighten the senses and make sure that the nervous system is constantly aware of everything that's going on, inside and outside the body, so that it can react appropriately.

For greater inner strength

With the mind sorted out, the nerves are happy to return to their natural state, helped along by the massage of the spinal reflexes (steps 29–37), which either placates or excites the nerves, whilst, at the same time, relaxing or strengthening the muscles. It also eases overall tension, improves circulation, and augments the natural functioning of all the major organs.

Open avenues of expression

The recipient's head relies on their neck and throat for the exchange of vital life force energies, the clarity of which is influenced by the lymphatic system. Although this system effectively infiltrates the whole body, there is a concentration of these reflexes in their toe necks (steps 22–28), so milking these well relieves neck and throat tension. It also facilitates the exchange of vital life forces and opens up avenues of expression.

Create inner harmony

The well-placed endocrine glands, which are miniscule members of the body, depend on the blood to transport their hormones to the target glands. The endocrine system responds exceptionally well to reflexology because not only are the glands themselves massaged (steps 38–45), one by one, but also all the reflexes throughout both feet, which effectively enhances the blood flow and sorts out the target cells. This helps to balance mind, body and soul, for complete inner harmony and overall well-being.

Make it easier to breathe

Massaging the balls of the feet (steps 46–50), soothes the respiratory and cardiac systems, making it much easier to breathe. This, in turn, stabilizes and comforts the heart and regulates the blood flow. Self-esteem and self-worth are boosted and the true spirit has a chance of shining through.

Help food on its way

Stroking and stimulating the insteps has a direct effect on the digestive tract (steps 51–75), which makes it so much easier to take in and digest all that is going on in life. It nourishes the mind, body and soul, and ensures that everything and everybody is fully appreciated. This is perfect for forming and maintaining fulfilling relationships. Massaging the lower halves of the insteps also influences the upper parts of the urinary tract, as well as reproductive and excretory systems, which really helps to get things moving. The end result is the ability to completely re-energize and rejuvenate oneself.

Back to the roots

The skeletal and muscular systems, as well as the lower parts of the excretory and reproductive systems, are represented on the heels. Kneading these reflexes (steps 76–93) makes the whole body so much more relaxed and far more flexible, making it much easier to let go of worked through thoughts and emotions and move on. Being able to participate fully in life's circumstances, constantly fills the whole persona with renewed energy. This, in turn, continually revitalizes the mind, body and soul, so much so that each individual can grow into the person that they really wish to be, which makes them feel so much more secure and happier within themselves.

For the next leg

Always complete each reflexology session with a gentle, but invigorating, overall massage (steps 94–103) because, by now, the feet and body are so relaxed that they happily allow themselves to be stretched beyond self imposed limits, which then helps them have a broader outlook and a more affable and flexible approach to life

The cycles of life defy a linear approach to life.

Reflexology today and in the future

Reflexology was valued as a healing medium for many centuries, but became less popular during the scientific revolution around 300 years ago. It, like many other concepts that link mind, body and soul, was soon dismissed as being unscientific. The body then became treated as some kind of sophisticated machine that could only be serviced and maintained by highly trained, specialized personnel. With many losing touch with their true selves, as well as with their connection to the Universe, it became inevitable that 'dis-ease' and unrest would become increasingly widespread. The resultant panic and hysteria worldwide has resulted in an unhealthy obsession with materialism, which has led to intense boredom, extreme emptiness and utter frustration, all of which impoverish the mind, exhaust the body and depress the soul.

Masses are literally starving and depriving themselves of the deeper meaning of life, which cannot be found or proven through scientific research: it just is. The only proof that natural remedies, such as reflexology, work is the ongoing well-being of those who receive it.

Fortunately, there is renewed interest in these ancient healing practices, because many now realize, that solutions are not confined to the physical world alone. Although many people turn to reflexology as a last resort when all else has failed, they are constantly astounded at its effectiveness. They soon realize that inner peace and harmony are possible, even in these distressing times of violence, confusion and fear.

With more and more people taking responsibility for their health and wellbeing, not only do they heal themselves but they play a vital role in healing the whole world. Reflexology has a huge role to play in the future, which it is more than capable of doing. With reflexology, we as individuals will get better at being ourselves, as we improve every step of the way.

There is inside you, all of the potential that you wish to be,
All the energy to do whatever you would like to do,
If you imagine yourself as you would like to be, doing what you wish to do,
And every day take a step towards your dream,
Although at times it may seem impossible to hold onto that dream,
One day you shall awake to find that you are the person that you dreamed of,
Doing what you wish to do, simply because you had the courage
To believe in your potential and hold onto your dream!

taking it further

The author, Chris Stormer, is a world acclaimed authority on reflexology and is affectionately known worldwide as 'The Universal Foot Lady'. Her previous books are enjoyed by those with a general interest in this fascinating form of healing; they are also used as text and handbooks in reflexology and healing establishments throughout the world. There is also a comprehensive range of charts, DVDs, videos, audio tapes available which can be viewed on www.alwaysb.com

Contacts, reflexology centres and training organizers

Book list

Refer to 'The Larkin List of Reflexology Books' – the most comprehensive list of reflexology books:

http://homepage.e ircom.net/~footman/

The Language of the Feet, also written by Chris Stormer provides some fascinating insight, as well as some deeper understanding, of the ever-changing characteristics of the feet. With life being constantly on the move, and needs constantly changing, this book makes it so much easier to tune into individual needs since they can differ greatly from massage to massage!

Reflexology contacts

The author

Chris Stormer
Tel/fax: +27 (0) 11 803 9052
Mobile +27 (0) 82 855 4255
inspired@worldonline.co.za
www.alwaysb.com

Publications

Reflexology World Magazine,
PO Box 1032,
Bondi Junction, NSW 1355
Tel: +61 (0) 2 9300 9391
Fax: +61 (0) 2 9300 9216
Publisher: Russell McAllister
reflexologyworld@yahoo.com.au

World Organization ICR
www.icr.reflexology.org

Specialized reflexology

AURA-SOMA® Colour reflexology – New Zealand

Janice Hill
Tel: +64 (0) 6 357 9318
Fax: +64 (0) 6 357 9338
janice.hill@xtra.co.nz
www.colourconnections.co.nz

Chi reflexology – Australia

Moss Arnold
Tel: +61 (0) 2 4754 5500
Fax: +61 (0) 2 4754 5588
info.@chi-reflexology.com.au
www.chi-reflexology.com.au

Colour reflexology – United Kingdom
Pauline Wills
Tel/fax: +44 (0))20 8204 7672
info@oracleschoolofcolour.com
www.oracleschoolofcolour.com

Ayuvedic reflexology – Australia
Sharon Strathis
Tel: +61 (0) 7 3878 1471
Fax: +61 (0) 7 3378 7514
info@ayurvedicreflexology.com
www.ayuvedicreflexology.com

Reflexology – workshops and information

OK in HEALTH website:
www.OKinHealth.com
Canada, USA, UK, Ireland

Reflexology associations

America

Maine Council of Relexologists
PO Box 5538
Augusta
ME4330-5583
info@maonline.org
www.reflexologyofmaine.org

NY State Reflexology
Association
Tel: +1 914 472 2521
president@nysraweb.org

Reflexology Association of
America
Tel: +1 740 657 1695
Fax: +1 740 657 1695
raaadminsupport@aol.com

Reflexology Association of
California
Tel: +1 562 433 3595
RACCalifornia@aol.com

Arizona
Jocelyn Ross Shields
Tel: +1 (602) 867-3717
JShields18@cox.net

New Jersey
Elaine Gorden
elainegorden@vzavenue.net

Massachusetts
Ginny Hahn
Massachusetts Association of
Reflexology
+1 508 423 9031
hahngin@comcast.net

Rhode Island
Margo Dussault
Tel: +1 401 423 1575
Fax: +1 401 864 0859
margod@naisp.net

Washington state
Shellie Earley
Tel: +1 (360) 513 7745
shelliesessentialoils@yahoo.com

Australia

Reflexology Association of Australia
Emma Gierschick – President
Tel: + 61 (0) 3 9774 3776
innasoul@optusnet.com.au
www.innasoul.com.au

Adelaide
Joyce Lockett
Tel: +61 (0) 8 8276 3547
joylock@picknowl.com.au

Susan Jean Ramsey
Tel: +61 (0) 8 8449 7091 –
Semaphore
Tel: +61 (0) 8 8626 1683 –
Streaky Bay
sjramsey@chariot.net.au

Brisbane
Jan Williams
Tel: +61 (0) 7 3272 4078
janwilliams29@hotmail.com

Melbourne
Australian School of
Reflexology and Relaxation
Tel: +61(0)3 9898 1890
Fax: +61(0)3 9898 1810
info@asrr.com.au
www.asrr.com.au

Perth
Joan Cass
Tel/fax: 61 (0)8 9354 5403
joancass@bigpond.com

Sydney
Sue Ehinger
The Australian School of
Reflexology
Tel: +61 (0)2 4976 3881
Fax: +61 (0) 2 49440 0906
reflexologyaustralia@gmail.com

Tasmania
Kaylene Archer
larcher@tassie.net.au

Canada

International Institute of
Reflexology
iircanada@sympatico.ca

Okanagan, BC
Maria Carr
Tel: + 1 250 492 4759
Mar-car@shaw.ca
www.OKinHealth.com

Toronto
Cathy Biedinger
Tel: +1 519 442 7383
iam2@execulink.com

Vancouver
Margo Nielsen
Tel: + 1 604 589 3599
Fax: + 1 778 828 8005
healthyenergy@shaw.ca

Vernon
Gwen Miller
Tel: + 1 (0) 250-545-7063
gwen_miller@telus.net

New Zealand

Xanthe Ashton
President, Reflexology NZ
xanthe@reflexology.co.nz
www.reflexology.org.nz

South Africa

The South African
Reflexology Society
Tel: 021 558 9868
Fax: 088 021 588 9868
info@sareflexology.org.za

Cape Town

Andrea Meyer
Tel: +27 (0) 21-701 3995
soletherapy@intekom.co.za

Durban

Yavanee Singh
Tel/fax: +27 (0)31 3120881
yavanee@absamail.co.za

Johannesburg

Keith McFarlane
Tel: +27 (0) 11 682 3584
RHASA@global.co.za

Sarisha M Harilal
Tel: +27 (0) 11 807 7365
sarisha@worldonline.co.za

Natal

Carol Francis
Tel: +27 (0) 33 997 0684
oroptimism@polka.co.za

South America

Rio De Janeiro

Sally Teixeira
Tel: +55 (0) 21 2522 1341
sally@reflexologyinrio.com

United Kingdom

Association of Reflexologists
Tel: +44 (0) 1823 351 010
Fax: +44 (0) 1823 336 646
info@aor.org.uk
www.aor.org.uk

British Reflexology
Association
Nicola Hall
Tel: +44 (0) 886 821207
Fax: +44 (0) 1886 822017
bra@britreflex.co.uk
www.britreflex.co.uk

England

Kent
Salvina B. Macari
'Empower Your Life'
Tel: + 44 (0) 1843 295910
Fax: +44 (0) 1843 294 778
salvinamacari@hotmail.com

Isle of Skye
John Cross
Tel: +44 (0) 1470 511 361
jrcacupressure@hotmail.com
www.johncrossclinics.com

Maidenhead
Ann Hodgson
Natural Therapies
Tel: +44 (0) 1628 621 157
a.hodgson247@btinternet.com

Norfolk
Angela Sellans Drake MAR
Pathways School of
Reflexology
Tel: +44 (0) 1603 503 794
Fax: +44 (0) 1603 457 331
asdrake@nthworld.com
www.pathwaysreflexology.co.uk

Ireland
The National Register of
Reflexologists
http://nationalreflexology.ie

County Roscommon
Anthony Smith
Little House of Avalon
Tel/fax: +353 (0) 905 83002
info@littlehouseofavalon.com
www.littlehouseofavalon.com

New Ross
Anthony Larkin
The European Institute of
Classical Reflexology
Tel: +353 51 422209
footman@eircom.net
http://homepage.eircom.net/~
footman/

Northern Ireland
Belfast
Kathy Green
Therapies Inc
Tel: +44 (0) 28 9029 5960
kathy.green@therapiesinc.co.uk
www.therapiesinc.co.uk

Coleraine
Sharon Johnston
Tel: +44 (0) 028207 42535
serenity04@btinternet.com
info@therapybysj.co.uk

Scotland
Edinburgh
Diane Scott
Tel: +44 (0) 131661 4150
Mob: + 44 (0) 7711 257 895
diinfeet@aol.com

South Lanarkshire
Sarah-fiona Helme
Tel: +44 (0) 1698 792768
sarahfionah@yahoo.com

Wales
Cardiff
Sue Evans
Tel: +44 (0)2920 512508
inspira1@btinternet.com

Pembrokeshire
Liz Evans
Tel: +44 (0) 1834 871 1402
footloos@talk21.com

appendix I

Healing enhanced through the use of oils

The sensuous aspect of aromatherapy oils has a therapeutic effect on mind, body and soul. A mixture of one to three oils, within approximately 30 mls of base oil, rubbed into the feet, at the end of a reflexology session, really enhances its affects. There are six main types of oils.

Uplifting oils	Boost confidence, ease depression and eliminate moodiness. Examples include clary sage, jasmine and grapefruit.
Regulating oils	Relieve anxiety and re-establish equilibrium. Examples include bergamot, frankincense, geranium and rosewood.
Stimulating oils	Strengthen concentration, clear the mind and improve memory. Examples include lemon, peppermint, rosemary and black pepper.
Invigorating oils	Fill the whole being with enthusiasm and interest, thereby strengthening the immune system. Examples include cardamom, juniper, rosemary and lemongrass.
Soothing oils	Increase levels of tolerance, improve sleep patterns and calm the mind. Examples include camomile, lavender, marjoram and orange blossom.
Aphrodisiac oils	Strengthen relationships and boost self-esteem. Example are clary sage, patchouli and ylang ylang.

There are many other incredible aromatherapy oils, information on which can be obtained from a vast range of specialized books.

The vibration of colours for inner harmony

Visualization of colours during reflexology alters the vibrational tone of the healing energies, which are absorbed into the body, to fine-tune mind, body and soul and, in so doing, harmonize them as one for overall balance. The following guide suggests which colours to visualize but, should another colour come to mind, then use that colour instead.

Red	Fifth toes and heels	Provides security, mobility and enthusiasm for ongoing development. 'See red' when things get in the way of one's progress.
Orange	Fourth toes and lower halves of instep	Communicates the joy of feeling secure in one's relationships, which makes life such a pleasure.
Yellow	Third toes and upper halves of insteps	Provides the passion to instigate ideas and make them a reality.
Green	Second toes and balls of the feet	Harmonizes the internal and external environments, creating space in which to be oneself.
Blue	Toe necks	Clears the way for the exchange of life force energies, closing the gap between the physical and non-physical.

Purple	All toes	By clearing the mind, it provides space in which to think and to find an inner peace and balance by reconnecting with the Divine source.

Music to relax the body, mind and soul

There's a huge section of the most incredible music that is ideal to use alongside reflexology. The following are a few suggestions to help you on your way.

Dolphin and whale music	Particularly beneficial during pregnancy and childbirth, as well as for special needs children and for disturbed, restless souls.
Natural sounds	Such as wind, birdsong, waterfalls, and waves. Example are: *Wilderness* by Tony O'Conner *Wetland Symphony* by Ducks Unlimited, Canada
Ethnic music	Using traditional instruments such as drums, didgeridoos, panflutes and so on. Example include: *Eagle* by Medwin Goodall *Uluru* by Tony O'Connor
Electric harp	An example is: *Dream spiral* by Hilary Stagg
Others	*Gifts of the Angels* by Steven Halpern *Bushman dreaming* by Tony O'Connor *Inner tides* by Ian Cameron Smith

appendix IV

Getting on the nerves

	Irritability	Tolerance	Patience	Sensitivity
too much	Sets the 'nerves on edge'.	The 'dis-ease' to please causes inner antagonism and suppressed ill feelings towards others.	Endurance and persistence that test patience until you can't take any more and snap.	Overly concerned and anxious from getting too involved, with the tendency to over-react to the slightest thing and take umbrage.
too little	Numbness or paralysis from 'deadening the nerves' so that it's no longer possible to feel the pain of the memory.	Complete intolerance, which usually comes out in an allergic reaction.	Impatience leading to edginess and agitation.	Appear indifferent, unresponsive, cold or unconcerned as a form of protection because of so much upset and hurt in the past.

Achilles pull 156–7
Achilles stretch 157
acupressure and acupuncture 10
adolescents 18
adrenal dis–order 96
adrenal gland reflexes 96–7, 112, 182
adulthood 18–19
advantages of learning reflexology 3–4
after-effects of reflexology 143
airway reflexes 79
Alexander technique 9
anal reflex 190
angles of feet 40
ankle reflexes 67
anus reflexes 124, 200
appendix reflexes 108–9
arches 53, 56
aromatherapy 10, 148, 230
ascending colon reflex 109–10, 196

babies 17–18, 99, 109, 110, 135
    and pregnancy 17, 127, 131–5, 209,
    233
back and limb reflexes 31–2
balls of the feet 69–86
    benefits of massage 84
    colour visualization 74–5, 231
    reflexes
    airways 73, 79
    breast 28, 73, 76
    elbow 79
    knees 80
    lungs 75
    oesophagus 73, 78
    pyloric sphincter 99
    ribcage 73, 82
    sensory system 60–1
    solar plexus 81
    thymus gland 73, 77
    upper arms 113
    upper back 83
benefits of reflexology 3–4
big toes 57–61
    hormones 59

natural characteristics 58–9
    sensory system 60–1
    reflexes
bladder reflexes 113, 124–5, 211
brain reflexes 42, 45, 54, 172
breast reflexes 27, 76–7, 205
breasts 27, 28, 70, 185
breathe and relax 152–3
buttock reflexes 122–3, 207

cancer 73, 74
cardiac sphincter reflexes 97
cardiac system reflexes 184
caterpillar movement 137, 138, 173
chest 28, 59, 70, 73, 76, 84, 169
childbirth, reflexology during and after
    134–5, 202
childhood, benefits of reflexology 17–18
circulatory dis-eases 85
colour visualization 10, 39, 231
    see also skin colour
complementary steps 9–10
crystals 10

deep vein thrombosis 17
defusing distress 2, 19
descending colon reflex 109
digestive reflexes 115
digestive system 187–202
dis-ease 9–10, 11–15
distress, defusing 2, 19
distressed reflexes 150
duodenum reflex 99–100

ear reflexes 90
ease or disease 11–15
elbow reflexes 79–80
endocrine gland reflexes 150, 178, 179
energy centres 218
energy flow, opening 160–2, 178–9
excretory reflexes 112–3
excretory system 221
eye reflexes 72–3, 163, 180

facial lymphatic reflexes 64–5
fallopian tubes reflexes 111–2, 208–9
families, benefits of reflexology for 20
feather-stroke 139–40
feet reflexes 55–6
finale 213–18
first-aid reflexology 218
flat feet 53
flower remedies (Rescue Remedy) 10, 218
forehead reflexes 45–6

gall bladder reflex 93–4
Garfield, James, President of the United
    States 6

hair reflexes 44–5
hand reflexes 54–5
head reflexes 45–6
healing through your hands 35
heart reflexes 84–5
heels 116–30
    altered states 118
    colour visualization 118, 231
    reflexes
        anus 124
        bladder 124–5
        buttocks 122–3
        hip 122
        lower back 129–30
        male reproductive 128
        pelvic bone 121
        rectum 123
        testes 129
        urethra 125–6
        vagina 127–8
hepatic flexure reflex 197
herbs 10
Higher Self, connecting with the 58
hip reflexes 122
Hippocrates 8
history and background 4–5
homeopathy 10
hypertension 13

ileo-caecal valve reflex 107–8
inner aspects of the feet 125, 208
insteps 87–115
    colour visualization 88, 231
    reflexes
        adrenal gland 96–7
        appendix 108–9
        ascending colon 109
        cardiac sphincter 97
        descending colon 109
        digestive 91–2
        duodenum 99–100
        ears 90
        excretory 112
        fallopian tubes 111–12, 115
        gall bladder 93
        ileo-caecal valve 107–8
        jejunum 100
        kidney 104

liver 92–3
lumber vertebrae 114
middle back 101
mouth 105
nose 89–90
ovaries 110–11
pancreatic 94–5
pregnancy 127
pyloric sphincter 99
sigmoid colon 199
sigmoid flexure 199
small intestine 106–7
spleen 95–6
splenic flexure 198
stomach 98
transverse colon 109, 197
ureter 113
uterus 127

Japanese mythology 4–5
jaw reflexes 118–19
jejunum reflex 100, 194

kidney reflexes 112–3, 211
knee reflexes 80–1

large intestine reflexes 109–10
left foot 28, 40
liver reflexes 92–3
lower arm reflexes 82–3
lower back reflexes 129–130
lower torso reflexes 216
lumber vertebrae reflexes 114
lung reflexes 75
lymphatic system 46, 58, 220

male reproductive reflexes 128
massage technique 136–40
    caterpillar movement 138
    effects of 142, 143
    feather–stroke or healing procedure
        139–40
    rotation technique 137
    stroking or milking 138–9
    therapeutic benefits of 143–4
massage order 151–218
medicine, modern medicine and
    reflexology 8–9
Metamorphic technique 176–7
midbrain reflexes 45, 52, 172
middle back reflexes 101
milking 138–9
mind, your state of 41–7
mouth reflexes 105–6
muscular system 117, 221
music 10, 147, 148, 233

neck and throat dis-orders 64
nervous dis-orders 53, 59
nervous system 54, 56, 150, 160, 178,
    220
nose reflexes 89–90

oesophagus reflexes **73, 78–9, 191**
outer aspects of the feet **32**
ovaries reflexes **110–11**

pancreatic reflexes **94–5**
pelvic bone reflexes **121**
pigeon-toed **140**
pineal gland reflexes **72–3**
pituitary gland reflexes **59–60**
pregnancy **17, 127, 131–5, 209, 233**
  pregnant reflexes **132–4**
preparation **146–50**
  explanation of reflexology **148**
  foot bath **149**
  making the client comfortable **149**
pyloric sphincter reflexes **99**

quick massage **218**

rectum reflexes **123**
reiki **10**
reproductive system **104, 221**
  lower reproductive reflexes **126**
Rescue Remedy **10, 218**
respiratory problems **76**
rib reflexes **82**
right foot **28, 40**
rotation technique **137**

self-esteem **9, 70, 85, 184, 221**
sensations experienced during massage
  142
sensory reflexes **60–1**
shiatsu **10**
shin reflexes **83**
shoulder reflexes **66**
sigmoid colon reflex **109, 199**
sigmoid flexure reflex **199**
sinus reflexes **44–5**
skeletal reflexes **119–20, 221**
  disorders **118**
skin colour **6**
skin condition **49–50**
small intestine reflexes **100, 106–7, 194–5**
solar plexus reflexes **81, 177**
spinal reflexes **52, 158–9, 173**
  massaging **173, 220**
  rubbing **158–9**
spine, strengthen **173**
spine, stretch **214**
spleen reflex **95–6**
splenic flexure **198**
stomach reflexes **98**
Stormer, Chris, *The Language of the Feet*
  224
strokes **172, 173**
stroking (milking) **137, 138–9**

tension
  dissipation of through reflexology **24**
testes reflexes **129**
throat reflexes **63, 191**
thymus gland reflexes **77–8**

thyroid gland reflexes **65**
toe nails **46**
toe necks **57–61**
  benefits of massage **58**
  colour visualization **58, 64, 231**
  reflexes
    neck **168, 170**
    oesophagus **78–9**
    shoulder **66, 169**
    throat **63, 167**
    thyroid gland **65**
toes **57–60, 69–129**
  benefits of massage **58**
  colour visualization **58, 231**
  fourth toes **43–4, 104**
  little toes **117**
  and the Metamorphic technique **176**
  natural state of **47, 58–9**
  opening the energy flow **160–1**
  reconnecting with the Higher Self **58**
  reflexes
    back of head and neck **46**
    brain **42, 44–5**
    ears **90**
    eyes **72**
    facial lymphatic **64–5**
    forehead **45**
    jaw **118**
    mouth **105**
    nose **89–90**
    pituitary gland **59**
    spine **52**
    second toes **70**
    shape **49**
    size **49**
    skin condition **49–50**
    stature of **47**
    third toes **87–102**
  see also big toes
transverse colon reflexes **109**

ulcers **13**
unusual reactions to reflexology **144–5**
upper arm reflexes **113–4**
upper back reflexes **84, 174**
upper body flexing **215**
upper thoracic vertebrae **83–4**
ureter reflexes **113**
urethra reflexes **125–6, 212–3**
uterus reflexes **127, 209**

vagina reflexes **127–8**
vertebral reflexes **52, 83–4, 114**

warm-up **152**
witches **5**
wrist reflexes **66–7**

teach®
yourself

From Advanced Sudoku to Zulu, you'll find everything you need in the **teach yourself** range, in books, on CD and on DVD.

Visit **www.teachyourself.co.uk** for more details.

Bridge
British Empire, The
British Monarchy from Henry VIII, The
Buddhism
Bulgarian
Business Chinese
Business French
Business Japanese
Business Plans
Business Spanish
Business Studies
Buying a Home in France
Buying a Home in Italy
Buying a Home in Portugal
Buying a Home in Spain
C++
Calculus
Calligraphy
Cantonese
Car Buying and Maintenance
Card Games
Catalan
Chess
Chi Kung
Chinese Medicine
Christianity
Classical Music
Coaching
Cold War, The
Collecting
Computing for the Over 50s
Consulting
Copywriting
Correct English
Counselling
Creative Writing
Cricket
Croatian
Crystal Healing
CVs
Czech
Danish
Decluttering
Desktop Publishing
Detox

Digital Home Movie Making
Digital Photography
Dog Training
Drawing
Dream Interpretation
Dutch
Dutch Conversation
Dutch Dictionary
Dutch Grammar
Eastern Philosophy
Electronics
English as a Foreign Language
English for International Business
English Grammar
English Grammar as a Foreign Language
English Vocabulary
Entrepreneurship
Estonian
Ethics
Excel 2003
Feng Shui
Film Making
Film Studies
Finance for Non-Financial Managers
Finnish
First World War, The
Fitness
Flash 8
Flash MX
Flexible Working
Flirting
Flower Arranging
Franchising
French
French Conversation
French Dictionary
French Grammar
French Phrasebook
French Starter Kit
French Verbs
French Vocabulary
Freud
Gaelic

Gardening
Genetics
Geology
German
German Conversation
German Grammar
German Phrasebook
German Verbs
German Vocabulary
Globalization
Go
Golf
Good Study Skills
Great Sex
Greek
Greek Conversation
Greek Phrasebook
Growing Your Business
Guitar
Gulf Arabic
Hand Reflexology
Hausa
Herbal Medicine
Hieroglyphics
Hindi
Hindi Conversation
Hinduism
History of Ireland, The
Home PC Maintenance and
  Networking
How to DJ
How to Run a Marathon
How to Win at Casino Games
How to Win at Horse Racing
How to Win at Online Gambling
How to Win at Poker
How to Write a Blockbuster
Human Anatomy & Physiology
Hungarian
Icelandic
Improve Your French
Improve Your German
Improve Your Italian
Improve Your Spanish
Improving Your Employability

Indian Head Massage
Indonesian
Instant French
Instant German
Instant Greek
Instant Italian
Instant Japanese
Instant Portuguese
Instant Russian
Instant Spanish
Internet, The
Irish
Irish Conversation
Irish Grammar
Islam
Italian
Italian Conversation
Italian Grammar
Italian Phrasebook
Italian Starter Kit
Italian Verbs
Italian Vocabulary
Japanese
Japanese Conversation
Java
JavaScript
Jazz
Jewellery Making
Judaism
Jung
Kama Sutra, The
Keeping Aquarium Fish
Keeping Pigs
Keeping Poultry
Keeping a Rabbit
Knitting
Korean
Latin
Latin American Spanish
Latin Dictionary
Latin Grammar
Latvian
Letter Writing Skills
Life at 50: For Men
Life at 50: For Women

Life Coaching
Linguistics
LINUX
Lithuanian
Magic
Mahjong
Malay
Managing Stress
Managing Your Own Career
Mandarin Chinese
Mandarin Chinese Conversation
Marketing
Marx
Massage
Mathematics
Meditation
Middle East Since 1945, The
Modern China
Modern Hebrew
Modern Persian
Mosaics
Music Theory
Mussolini's Italy
Nazi Germany
Negotiating
Nepali
New Testament Greek
NLP
Norwegian
Norwegian Conversation
Old English
One-Day French
One-Day French – the DVD
One-Day German
One-Day Greek
One-Day Italian
One-Day Portuguese
One-Day Spanish
One-Day Spanish – the DVD
Origami
Owning a Cat
Owning a Horse
Panjabi
PC Networking for Small
  Businesses

Personal Safety and Self
  Defence
Philosophy
Philosophy of Mind
Philosophy of Religion
Photography
Photoshop
PHP with MySQL
Physics
Piano
Pilates
Planning Your Wedding
Polish
Polish Conversation
Politics
Portuguese
Portuguese Conversation
Portuguese Grammar
Portuguese Phrasebook
Postmodernism
Pottery
PowerPoint 2003
PR
Project Management
Psychology
Quick Fix French Grammar
Quick Fix German Grammar
Quick Fix Italian Grammar
Quick Fix Spanish Grammar
Quick Fix: Access 2002
Quick Fix: Excel 2000
Quick Fix: Excel 2002
Quick Fix: HTML
Quick Fix: Windows XP
Quick Fix: Word
Quilting
Recruitment
Reflexology
Reiki
Relaxation
Retaining Staff
Romanian
Running Your Own Business
Russian
Russian Conversation

Russian Grammar
Sage Line 50
Sanskrit
Screenwriting
Second World War, The
Serbian
Setting Up a Small Business
Shorthand Pitman 2000
Sikhism
Singing
Slovene
Small Business Accounting
Small Business Health Check
Songwriting
Spanish
Spanish Conversation
Spanish Dictionary
Spanish Grammar
Spanish Phrasebook
Spanish Starter Kit
Spanish Verbs
Spanish Vocabulary
Speaking On Special Occasions
Speed Reading
Stalin's Russia
Stand Up Comedy
Statistics
Stop Smoking
Sudoku
Swahili
Swahili Dictionary
Swedish
Swedish Conversation
Tagalog
Tai Chi
Tantric Sex
Tap Dancing
Teaching English as a Foreign
    Language
Teams & Team Working
Thai
Theatre
Time Management
Tracing Your Family History
Training

Travel Writing
Trigonometry
Turkish
Turkish Conversation
Twentieth Century USA
Typing
Ukrainian
Understanding Tax for Small
    Businesses
Understanding Terrorism
Urdu
Vietnamese
Visual Basic
Volcanoes
Watercolour Painting
Weight Control through Diet &
    Exercise
Welsh
Welsh Dictionary
Welsh Grammar
Wills & Probate
Windows XP
Wine Tasting
Winning at Job Interviews
Word 2003
World Cultures: China
World Cultures: England
World Cultures: Germany
World Cultures: Italy
World Cultures: Japan
World Cultures: Portugal
World Cultures: Russia
World Cultures: Spain
World Cultures: Wales
World Faiths
Writing Crime Fiction
Writing for Children
Writing for Magazines
Writing a Novel
Writing Poetry
Xhosa
Yiddish
Yoga
Zen
Zulu